Angels Among Us

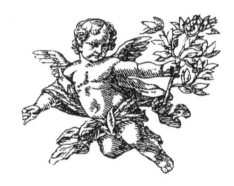

"Take the first step in faith. You don't have to see
the whole staircase, just the first step."
— Dr. Martin Luther King, Jr.

100% of the net royalties from the sale of this book are donated to Children's Hospitals.

All rights reserved under International and Pan-American copyright conventions.
Published in the United States by LifeSkills Press, Bainbridge Island, Washington, a division of
The Roots & Wings Society.

Printed in the USA on acid-free recycled paper
Library of Congress Cataloging-in-Publication Data Pending
ISBN 1-887703-01-2

Angels Among Us by the Real Santa Claus/Phil Smart, Sr.

Cover Art/Cheri Streimikes & Alison Asher
Portraits/Cheri Streimikes

All Photographs/Cynthia Becker White

Copyright 2001, LifeSkills Press a division of the Roots & Wings Society
Based upon stories submitted by Phil Smart, Sr.

The Roots & Wings Society, PO Box 11808, Bainbridge Island, Washington 98110
www.roots-wings.com

For my wife, Helen. . .

*Without my precious Helen by my side, these past sixty years,
my life could well have been devoid of real purpose.*

Thank you Sweetheart, for everything.

IV

TABLE OF CONTENTS

Children's Hospital we know today. That is because I have written the following as a child's version of the story of Anna Clise and all the volunteers who have given their love and lives to Children's Hospital.

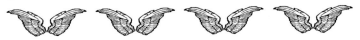

Once upon a time, in a forest by the sea, there lived a woman whose name was Anna.

Anna was very, very sad. She had a son who was the light of her life. When he was sad, she was sad. When he smiled, she smiled — So much so that even the angels were jealous.

One day the boy got very sick and Anna could not make him smile again. Alas, despite all she could do, all anyone could do, he journeyed on to heaven. The angels rejoiced to have another angel in their midst. But Anna was very, very sad.

Then one day, she was walking by the sea and came upon an oyster. The oyster said, "Why are you so sad?" And so she told him.

"Well," said the oyster, "Within my shell I have many difficulties — irritations, you know — things that chafe and hurt and will not go away. But I have learned a secret. If you dream, and if you work very hard, you can make a thing of beauty from your sadness... a pearl of great value."

And on that day Anna declared that she would make a pearl. Her pearl would be a little house of healing for children only. Where mothers with children whose smiles had gone away could go to get their smiles back.

She called all the other mothers together and they agreed to help. They got very busy. And the men helped too. By and by, there was a cottage on the hill where the fresh air blew, where children found their smiles again.

And often, very often, miracles happened within those walls.

Through the generations, the cottage grew on the bounty of the town. And mothers who knew the lesson of the oyster came to the cottage to make pearls of their sadness and beacons of their hope.

Of course, sometimes there were storms and the winds of change blew cruel. But if the children had a need, it rained not cats and dogs, but pennies and dollars and all good things on the little house of healing. There was always enough — and just a little bit more— for the next stormy day that came their way.

And so it is that for generations children have come from near and far to a place where, every day, miracles happen.

And now, dear friends, it is up to you to see that for ages and ages, henceforth and evermore, there will always be a little house of healing for children only.

For now. . . Anna Clise's pearl is in your hands.

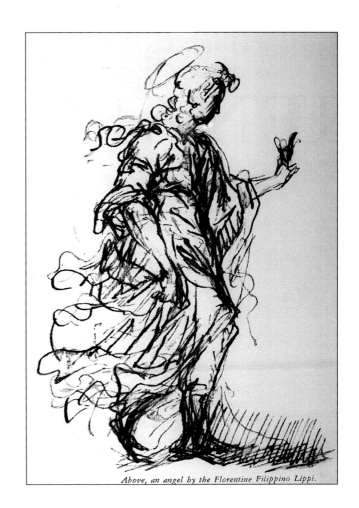

Above, an angel by the Florentine Filippino Lippi.

X

INTRODUCTION

by Mark Cutshall

Forty years ago, Phil Smart, Sr. made time in his crowded schedule for a five-minute appointment that changed his life forever. The receptionist at his dealership, Philip Smart Mercedes-Benz, said to him one morning, "There's a woman in the lobby waiting to see you. She says her name is Grandma Christmas Card."

"With a name like that," Phil recalls, "I knew she had to be in marketing." Her real name was Peg Emory, a volunteer with Children's Hospital. And within a few minutes she had persuaded the car dealer to buy several dozen engraved Christmas cards to support the hospital's work. But Peg wasn't through. A few days later, she returned to Phil's office with a personal invitation. "Since the hospital was founded in 1907, we've never had a man volunteer his time in the evenings to visit our young patients. The all-woman board of directors would like you to be that person. It would just be three hours, one night a week. Will you do it?"

"Where is the manual for male volunteers?" Phil asked. "We don't have one," said Peg. "Once you meet the children you won't need any instructions." With no formal training on how to comfort critically ill children and after assuring his wife that it would mean three hours one night a week, Phil said "yes" to Peg Emory's invitation.

That initial visit turned into three visits, and then six months of visits, and then a year. Soon, a lifetime of giving to others unfolded with no expectation other than the opportunity to share himself with the children who have taught him what life is all about. "For the past forty years, every Wednesday night, I have been able to go to this place I call 'The Miracle House' [Children's Hospital and Regional Medical Center]. It's been my school where I have learned about life. . . . Every visit, every child has become a precious gift unwrapped before me. . . ."

There was Bonnie, who as a ten-year-old could move only her head and tongue, but who found a way to earn both a bachelor's and master's degree in counseling so she could help drug addicts in her home town get back on their feet. And there was Jeff, who met Phil thirty-one years ago. Jeff came to the Miracle House to recover from a catastrophic injury. Today he too is a ward volunteer.

One day, the hospital called and offered Phil what he refers to as "a promotion." They asked him to donate more of his time. When he asked, "How much more time?" the voice on the other end of the line said, "Not much, just one additional day a year. We'll give you a new suit for the job. But you might not like the color. It's all red." Phil took his new job to heart and soon became affectionately known as "The Real Santa Claus." Phil is nearly eighty-two years old now. He has been a ward volunteer for more than half of his life. If ever there were a real Santa Claus who understands the gift of giving, you'll find him at the Miracle House every Wednesday night.

"I've had the privilege to know each of these children by name. I've shared their hopes and fears. They have shown me the one thing in life I could never have possibly understood on my own. That is, how a little time invested in another person can transform your heart. . . and change the world."

This is a lesson Phil had already learned as a Scoutmaster and past president of the Chief Seattle Council, and as a forty-one year member and past-president of Seattle "4" Rotary, the largest Rotary Club in the world. When he reports in for his weekly visits, some of the young patients call him the "angel from heaven." Phil chuckles and says, "I've never heard a car dealer called that before!"

While this book is his first attempt at telling his stories in print, Phil often speaks with large groups. Invariably, one universal question arises from the audience. "How do you run a business, deal with the demands of daily life, and find time to volunteer?" He smiles and says,

"I've been given as much time as anyone else — eight hours to work, eight hours to sleep, and eight hours to spend as I please. It's out of this 'third eight' that I've become a changed person. The children at the hospital have molded me into a happier man."

By this time Phil's audience is leaning forward as if to say, "Tell me more." He is grateful to oblige. He shares the stories of his young 'teachers' with his audience, hoping that a bit of his vision will rub off on them. Some are wiping their eyes. Some are smiling. All are listening.

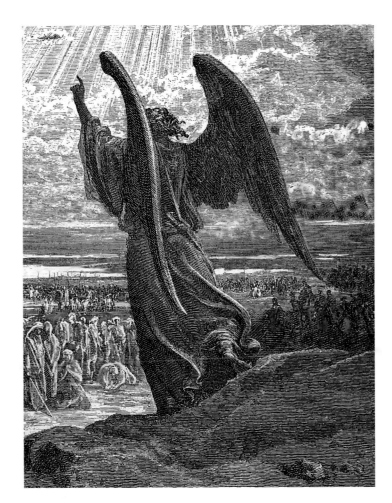

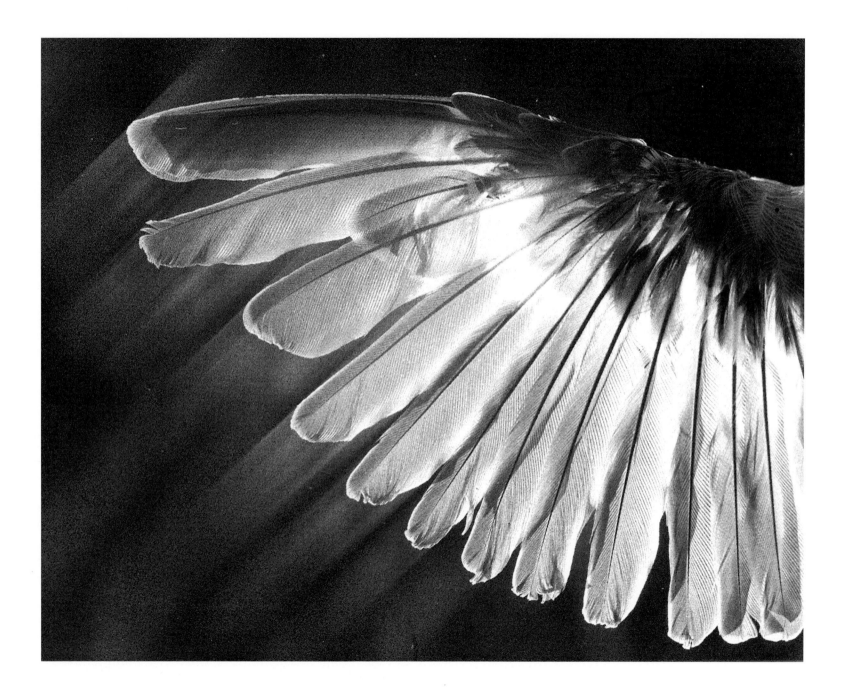

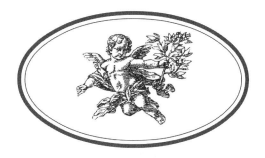

THE THIRD EIGHT

"We are like children who stand in need of masters to enlighten us and direct us, and God has provided angels to be our teachers and guides."
— Saint Thomas Aquinas

We all have the same twenty-four hours in each day, no more, no less. I have never met anyone, young or old, who has been blessed with twenty-five hours or cursed with twenty-three. No matter what our economic status may be, what language we speak, or what part of the world we may live in, we all have the same amount of time each day. Most of us work eight hours and sleep eight hours, which leaves a third eight hours in each of our days. It is how we use this *third eight* that defines the quality of our lives. We have to ask ourselves, how are we choosing to spend that most precious commodity, our time?

I was born and raised in Seattle, and I love my city dearly. I have seen it change dramatically over the years, from 1920 to the present day.

Yet throughout these many long years, I have noticed that eight areas of pain remain constant within the streets of my beloved city. These eight areas of pain are: the hurting, the hungry, the homeless, the unemployed, the drugged, the young, the old, and the illiterate.

It has also become clear to me that these eight areas of pain exist in every other city, town, and village in the world. In Los Angeles, London, Berlin, Cairo, Tokyo, Bethlehem, and Moscow, we all share the same areas of pain and the same number of hours in each day.

I have come to believe that the true measure of a life is not its duration, but its *donation*. You may believe that you cannot contribute a portion of your third eight hours. You may be saying to yourself "I don't have enough hours in the day as it is!" Perhaps you believe your time is not your own.

Some years ago, I chose to donate a piece of my third eight — just three hours a week — to the first area of pain, the hurting. In my case it was night school. The tuition was free: just a small investment of my time. My teachers were as abundant as they were diverse, from premature babies to young adults.

The subjects I studied were lessons in life, death, courage, determination, and victory. It was in this night school that I obtained my master's degree in faith, hope — and love.

My experience as a ward volunteer at Children's Orthopedic Hospital and Regional Medical Center has reshaped my life entirely. Certainly, each of us has three hours a week and our own particular calling to the young or the old, the hungry or the illiterate. You might say to yourself, *I don't do well with people who are hurting, and spending time with the elderly doesn't seem to fit either.* What area of pain is calling you? Can you imagine yourself helping someone else learn to read?

What do you think might happen if each of us, all over the world, gave a small piece of our third eight — our God-given talents, our energy, our courage, our empathy, our determination — to one of those areas of pain?

What do you think would happen? Well, in a very short period of time, I think we just might change the world.

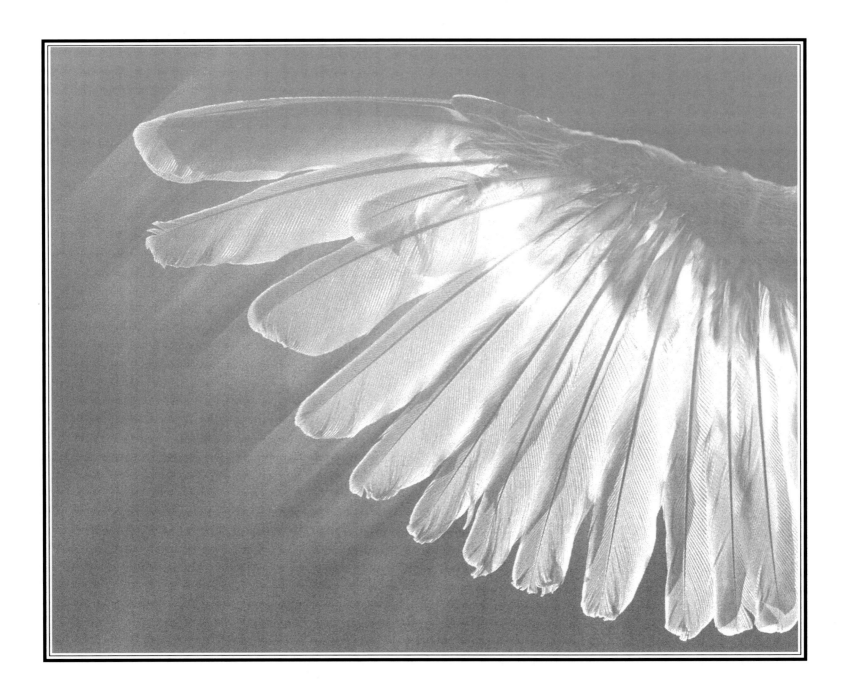

CHAPTER TWO – DARKNESS INTO LIGHT

"How do you be helpful to someone else who is worried? Well, here is an example: Friday at school is popcorn day. It costs 25 cents. So if somebody is sad, you can buy a large bag of popcorn for them as a present and you might have enough money left for yourself. But, I would also feel a bit sorry for myself if I didn't get any. But the louder voice inside of you says, *It was worth it.*"

—— Josh M. – 8 years old.

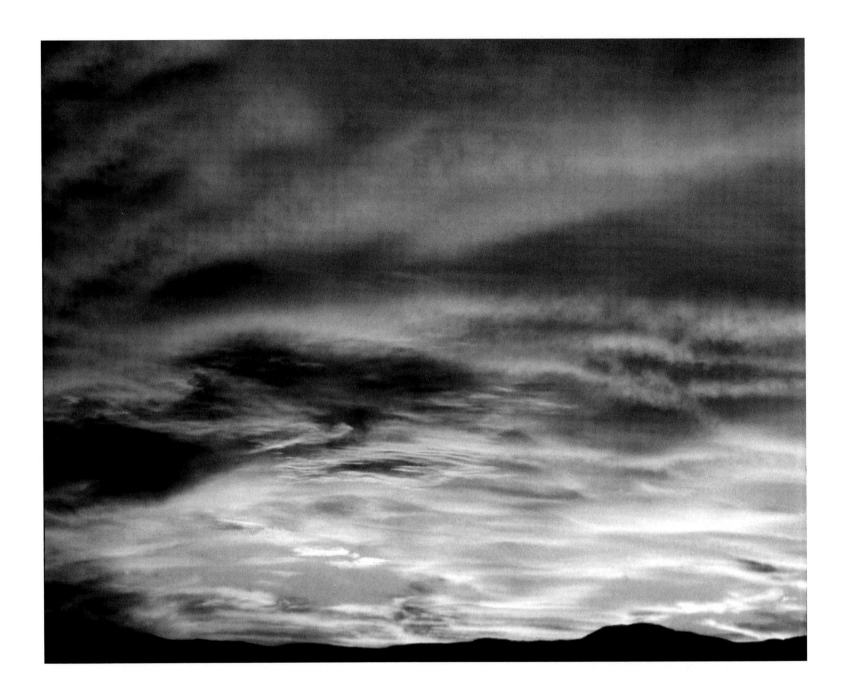

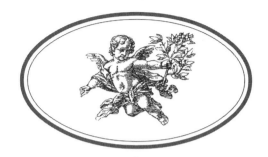

DARKNESS INTO LIGHT

"And the darkness turned into light and night into day..."
— Genesis

I hunched my shoulders further into my raincoat, bowed my head against the driving rain, and quickly made my way toward the warm glow of the entrance. This was the place. The plaque on the exterior wall confirmed it— blue and white, the babe in swaddling clothes, "Children's Orthopedic Hospital and Medical Center."

I went through the double swinging doors, past an empty wheelchair and up to the reception counter where a cheerful smile guided me on.

"The Volunteer Office is located one floor down, turn right as you exit the elevator."

I can still vividly recall the volunteer supervisor's instructions as she said, "Don't become emotionally involved with any of the patients.

It will be difficult to maintain an arm's length relationship, but that's how it must be, of course."

Once the instruction session was completed, I was assigned to One South, the teenage ward. An imposing sign on the wall escorted me into this remarkable adventure.

WASH YOUR HANDS BEFORE GOING INTO THE WARDS. SIGN IN AND OUT AND TOTAL YOUR HOURS AFTER EACH EVENING'S ASSIGNMENT.

The children were twelve to twenty years old but their wisdom far exceeded their actual ages. I entered their rooms tentatively, believing *I* was there to entertain *them*. Yet, behind each door, I discovered a unique, loving, and vibrant soul whose eyes (like those of a teacher) seemed to silently say, "I see my student has arrived."

Once my rounds were complete that first night, I went to the elevator, pushed the UP button and then, impatient at the delay, walked up the two flights of stairs to the lobby. I bade the receptionists good night, "See you next week." I dodged a cab driver in the lobby who was hurriedly responding to a blood call, then pushed through the double doors. The moon was playing tag with fast moving clouds. The clear night air filled my lungs.

I backed my car from the parking space and drove off into the darkness.

And so the experience began, the years of excitement, anticipation, laughter, and tears; a kaleidoscope of emotions, a cornucopia of rewards, all under the antiseptic title of "Ward Volunteer."

Each child was different and yet somehow the same. Their family life, traditions, and ethnic individuality were tied together by strong common threads: compassion, understanding, patience, and love. They gave of themselves wholeheartedly to anyone with whom they had any contact, no matter how brief. These remarkable mentors offered lessons in living life abundantly and accepting death gracefully.

As the owner of a small car dealership, I had learned all the appropriate skills for success in the marketplace. I developed my order-asking and closing techniques, maintained a positive attitude with my customers, and honed my sales abilities. As a ward volunteer, the children taught me more enduring life-lessons.

During my time as a ward volunteer, the children have reshaped my soul and molded me into a new man. I learned unwavering determination and deep faith from Bonnie, genuine forgiveness from Lynn, loyalty from Jimmy, and true patience from Kathy. Billy taught me to be thankful for what I have, and Lisa taught me how to hug soul to soul.

Most entrepreneurs will tell you how nerve-racking owning a small business can be. The financial tides tend to ebb and flow, while the needs of the employees and their families remain constant. Playfulness and peace of mind are not the usual qualities one maintains under circumstances such as these.

Before I began consciously giving away my *third eight*, the vast majority of my time was spent hurrying from one task to another and worrying about the outcome of my efforts. Moments of playfulness and peace of mind were in the minority. Now, those ratios have been reversed completely.

If you listen carefully to the children whose life-lessons are chronicled within the pages of this book, their messages will stay with you forever. I must forewarn you that some of these stories end in death. But, as I have learned, they only appear to end there. In the beginning of my volunteer experience, I often drove home from the hospital pounding the steering wheel and repeatedly yelling, "Why?"

As time passed, I began to gain some peace with regard to that horrible question. I learned the difference between a broken heart and a broken spirit. I received this blessing while apprenticing with another amazing teacher. Her name was Lynn, and her story will come later.

It is difficult to comprehend the burdens some of these children carry. Yet their insights may influence you as they have me, if you come to understand the difference between having empathy and taking pity. I have found that pity is usually a misplaced emotion.

My wife, Helen, and I learned an extraordinary lesson while we were consoling a bereaved mother. She shared with us a vivid dream that forever altered her perspective on children with medical concerns. In her dream she saw these young ones as the wisest angels in heaven, carefully choosing their fate before arriving here on earth. Each one seemed to know how their sacrifice would serve to reshape the souls of those who loved them. This beautiful dream still stirs my heart.

Could it be that children who face physical challenges or whose lives are foreshortened have consciously chosen their fate? Why are so many of these children exceedingly patient and wise beyond their years? When looking into their eyes in the quiet moments I can't help but wonder, "Are these well developed souls who are wearing small disguises?" While I do not pretend to understand the mysteries of this life or the next, I have come to believe that we actually do have angels among us.

I would love to tell you each of their stories, but a book that size would be completely unmanageable. My editor has allowed me to include just a sampling of these experiences. Please come with me now as we visit just a few of these extraordinary teachers.

"Some people
come into
our lives
and quickly go.
Some stay for awhile
and leave
footprints on our
hearts.
And we are
never, ever the same."

— Albert Einstein

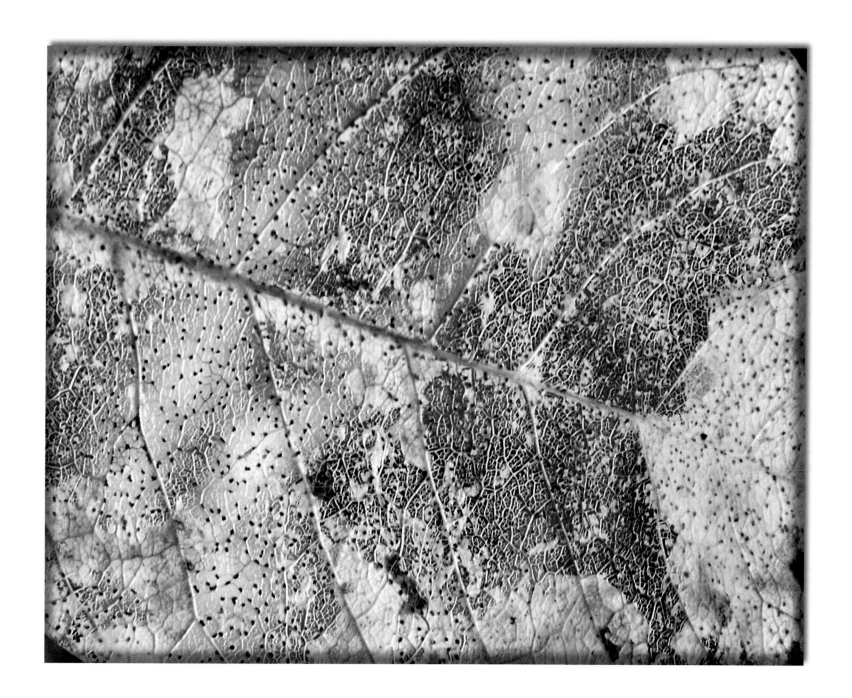

CHAPTER THREE ≈ HIDDEN BLESSINGS

"When someone you love is sick you feel upset. You might be afraid about what will happen to them. But it helps to pretend they are still nearby you, even if they are in the hospital faraway, because when some-body loves you, it's like they are right inside of you wherever you go."

— Bobby M. - 6 years old

"The greatest

good

you can do

for another

is not just share your

riches,

but reveal to them

their own."

—Benjamin Disraeli

While the staff was sadly aware of the reasons for the reunion, they were always happy to see their old friend Rosie. To know her was to love her; and once you did, you never wanted to let her go.

I remember one evening in particular when her room was crowded with family and friends. Holding court from her bedside, she flashed her bright smile and beckoned me in. Again, she was wearing a pair of outrageous knee socks. This time they were red, yellow and blue. Once I had settled into my chair, she asked me a startling question, "Did you know that I'm supposed to die in three weeks?" A hush fell over the room.

"No, I didn't," I answered.

"Well, I am. Do you believe it?" she inquired with intense concentration.

Looking into her big brown eyes I asked, "Do you believe it?"

"Oh yes," she quickly replied, "certainly."

I was baffled by this response. I wondered why this exuberant spirit wasn't willing to fight. Then I wondered if, perhaps, there was no need to fight at all. Some people have a deep knowing about when their time has come. Was this the case with Rosie? Either way, a thought came clearly to mind and I wanted to share it with her. "Rosie, will you do something for me?"

"Of course!" was her ready reply.

"Each night as you close your eyes I want you to take a deep breath, relax and say to yourself, 'All things are possible with God!' Will you do that?"

"Yes, I will," she promised.

Our eyes were riveted on one another. "Each morning as you awake, will you say the same thing?"

"Yes, yes." She spoke with certainty. We both began smiling. When I looked up I noticed that her friends were smiling as well.

The following Wednesday evening I brought an empty pad of paper to share with Rosie. I knocked on her door and was relieved to see that she did not have any visitors at the moment. She was braiding her hair when she looked up from the mirror and asked, "What are you going to do with that?"

I drew a line down the center of the paper. Making two columns I said, "Let's talk about your plans for the next years of your life. What are your dreams, ambitions and wishes? We'll put that list down on the left side of the tablet. You just say what is on your mind and I'll write it down for you."

"Okay, let's see. Hmmm. First I'm going to finish high school, then I'm going to become a manicurist to earn money for college."

"You're going to college?" I asked.

"I'm going to be a neurologist."

"Great! Tell me more about the things you're interested in."

"I love to sing, write poetry and perform in drama class. I especially love being with my friends."

The list on the left side of the page grew longer as her dreams unfolded. When we reached the second page, her energy began to wane.

She asked, "How about the other half of the paper? What goes there?"

"The other side is for the difficult things in your life. And if you don't mind, I've taken the liberty of filling that in."

I handed her the tablet and she read the right-hand side aloud, "It seems that Rosie has a physical challenge that is being addressed by the caring experts in this Miracle House."

She looked at me and asked, "Nothing else on that side?"

"I could only find one problem."

"Live as if you were to die tomorrow. Learn as if you were to live forever."

—Mahatma Gandhi

"It is a pretty good score if you take a look at it." I responded. "Fifteen to one!"

She studied the pad of paper intently. Then, in her animated and articulate manner, she began reading the list aloud — each line with increasing dramatic flair. I applauded her performance. She mimed taking a deep bow while sitting upright in her bed. Then she let out a sigh and her head plopped back down on the pillow. Her eyes grew heavy with sleep. I waved good-night with the tablet and she waved back. As I closed the door behind me I could hear a faint whispering, "All things are possible. . ."

Rosie has far exceeded her previous belief of having only three weeks to live and continues to plan for her future. She doesn't know how many days she has remaining on this earth—none of us do. Her focus on the calendar has changed. Rather than counting down the days to her departure, she diligently counts her blessings at the close of each day.

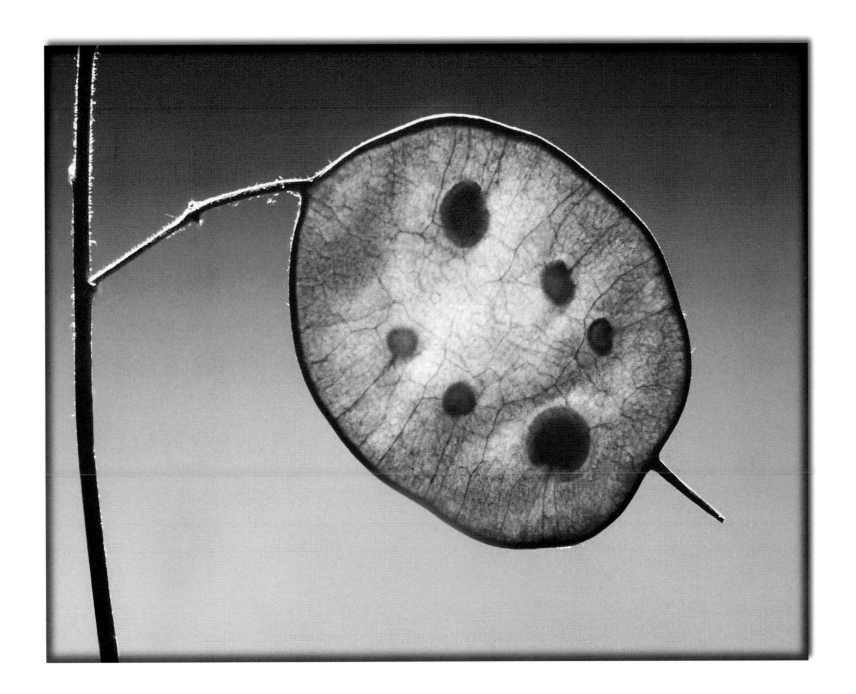

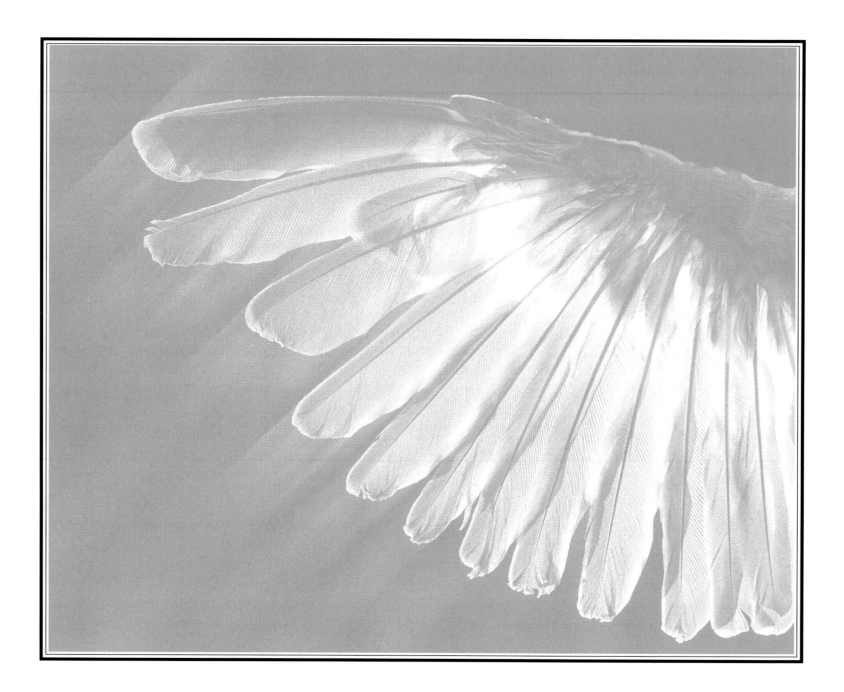

CHAPTER FOUR ~ THE RED SUIT

"But Mom, I don't want to leave the
hospital today even if it is Christmas.
The real Santa Claus comes here!"
— Connor age 6

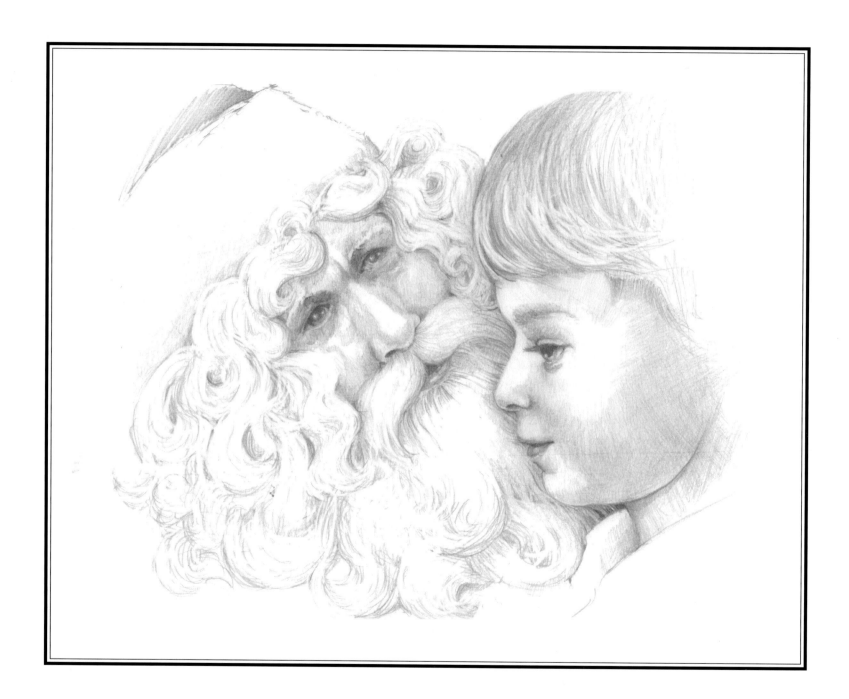

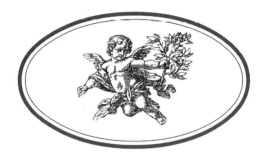

THE RED SUIT

"A dream is a private myth. A myth is a public dream."
— Joseph Campbell

Hanging in a wired enclosure for most of the year, it awaited a single magic day when it would again be put to use. The shiny black boots and large round sleigh bells rested in the cardboard box below it.

Removed from their musty storage on this special day, these items were transported to a huge building on a faraway hill. Soon, a thin man in a blue business suit would once again be transformed into a legend, just as he had every year for more than a quarter of a century. First came the dusting of eyebrows and lashes with chalk to emphasize age, and rouge to bring the color from the northern frost to his forehead, cheeks, and nose.

Then the binding of pillows around his middle created the familiar plump profile. The trousers and jacket trimmed in white were cinched firmly around his padded girth with a wide black belt. The soft flowing beard was affixed by bands around tender earlobes. With his wig carefully adjusted and his cap now in place at a jaunty angle, the transformation was complete.

As he stepped into the imposing hospital lobby, sleigh bells foretelling his entrance, the annual journey began. He had one hundred and twenty-seven stops to make. The red suit moved from one room to another, each one was different, yet somehow the same. There were smiles and tears, belief and disbelief. All cares and hurts were nearly forgotten as each child eagerly awaited a magical moment, a big hug and a small Christmas package. This was a day when the hospital walls could almost entirely disappear. Joy, anticipation, and the familiarity of family life filled the hallways before reality could return as an unwelcome guest.

"He's critical with leukemia, so don't tarry too long," whispered the duty nurse as Santa rounded the corner into the next room. The seven-year-old quietly shared his own conviction with Red Suit: "You know, what you have to have is good health, do as well as you can, and everything will turn out all right."

Mom closed her eyes and leaned into the soft white curls, seeking the comfort of a tender hug. He whispered a few words of reassurance, slowly walked to the door, and offered a farewell wave.

A young mother met him outside the next room. "She's not able to speak, even though she's seven." A beautiful child with blonde hair, blue eyes and a warm understanding smile awaited his entrance. Their heart-strings entwined as they savored their brief exchange. The conversation was one-sided, yet her eyes spoke clearly and lovingly.

At that moment, there came an interruption. An aide from the third floor appeared in the doorway and announced, "Sarah upstairs doesn't believe in you." In his haste, Red Suit nearly stumbled up the stairs to greet her. She was involved in a coloring project.

"Hi Sarah! I'm Santa Claus."

The beautifully freckled eight-year-old looked up from her artwork. "I don't believe in Christmas. I have Hanukkah!" Her father leaned over and said, "Shalom."

Santa replied, "Shalom to you, my friend. I know of the eight lights and the eternal tapers."

Moving on to the next child, Santa smiled to himself, recalling his warm relationship with the Senior Rabbi up the street. He turned to the woman standing by the bed.

"Are you her Mom?" he asked.

"Yes, she's mine. Eighteen years old with cystic fibrosis, and doing as well as we can expect."

He moved closer to the bedside, bent over the still figure entwined in tubes connected to machinery, and quietly spoke a word of faith. Memories of many answered prayers came to mind as he made his way to the next room.

A tender eight-year-old heart was mending. The vivid vertical line down the young boy's chest was mute testimony to the surgical expertise performed merely forty-eight hours earlier. "He's doing fine!" his mother exclaimed. The child's proud grin confirmed his mother's enthusiastic remark.

And so it went, hour after hour, a sharing of joys and sorrows, hopes and fears with Red Suit, a mysterious man who was unbelievable yet believable since here he was, as forecast and heralded.

As he moved through 3B, Oncology, he could never have known that a lifelong memory was about to unfold. Standing in the open doorway with a bag of gifts in hand, he awaited an invitation to enter.

"Lisa, Santa is here. Would you like to say hello?" Her reply was unheard, but Mom's comment was quite clear. "Come in Santa, she's feeling better now." The shades in the room were lowered. A tender darkness softened the morning light.

"Hi Lisa, I have some gifts for you. May I help you open one or two?"

A frail fourteen-year-old nodded yes. Her mouth was filled with shaved ice to soothe the aggravated sores on her tongue and cheeks. In violation of Miracle House rules, he sat next to her thin figure on the bed and placed a small gift in her hand.

Her response to the gift bordered on boredom. Suddenly she stretched out her arms to their limits and surprised him with a total embrace. As he began to gently pull away, the hug became more of a cling. He abandoned any notion of withdrawing, welcomed her gently into his soft white beard and wondered, "Could this moment have been heaven sent?"

Time stood still. No words were needed as he walked silently toward the door. With her strength waning, she smiled gently and waved good-bye.

He soon returned to 3B again, this time in a three-piece blue suit, raincoat over his arm and glasses in hand. A protective mother challenged him by quickly blocking the door. "Who are you?"

"I'm Santa. May I speak with Lisa?" He whispered so Lisa would not hear.

"Of course," Mom replied. "We wondered who you were. I apologize for being abrupt — you look so different. Before we go into her room I must tell you, I felt that something very special took place between you and Lisa. It happened during the hug she gave you. It was so unlike her to do something like that."

"I sensed the same thing; that's why I returned." They entered the room together.

"Lisa, this man wants to speak with you. Is that okay? "

Lisa fixed her eyes on him and spoke two words with clear recognition, "Santa Claus!"

Time stretched like warm taffy. They seemed to see each other soul to soul. Finally, he broke the silence and told her of his pending trip out of town. Making a note of two phone numbers, one for her room and the other for the care facility, he promised to call once he had arrived.

Later that night he leaned against the desk in the hotel lobby and listened impatiently to the repeated ringing at the other end of the line. Finally, an unfamiliar voice answered.

"May I speak with Lisa?"

"She isn't here."

"I'll call the other number, thank you."

"You won't reach her there either. She has passed away."

The words hung in the air like an unwelcome echo. A tremendous vacancy engulfed him. The clamor of the hotel lobby slowed and softened until there was only stillness. The hotel seemed to disappear completely. Then, as though it were actually happening again, he could feel Lisa's loving embrace pressing indelibly into his heart.

The images of the children rolled over and over in his mind. He could see them all, from fragile one-and-a-half pound premature babies to high-spirited young adults. Some were newly adjusting to their confining circumstances while others were veterans of long-term care. Yet all of them were wanting the same things: courage, understanding, pain relief, and recovery.

Santa had listened to each of them, sensed the unspoken and at the visit's end, removed the vestiges of the day. He carefully put them away until another year would pass. Certainly the teardrops on the red suit would have dried by then.

"Let the tears flow of their own accord; their flowing is not inconsistent with inward peace and harmony."

— Seneca

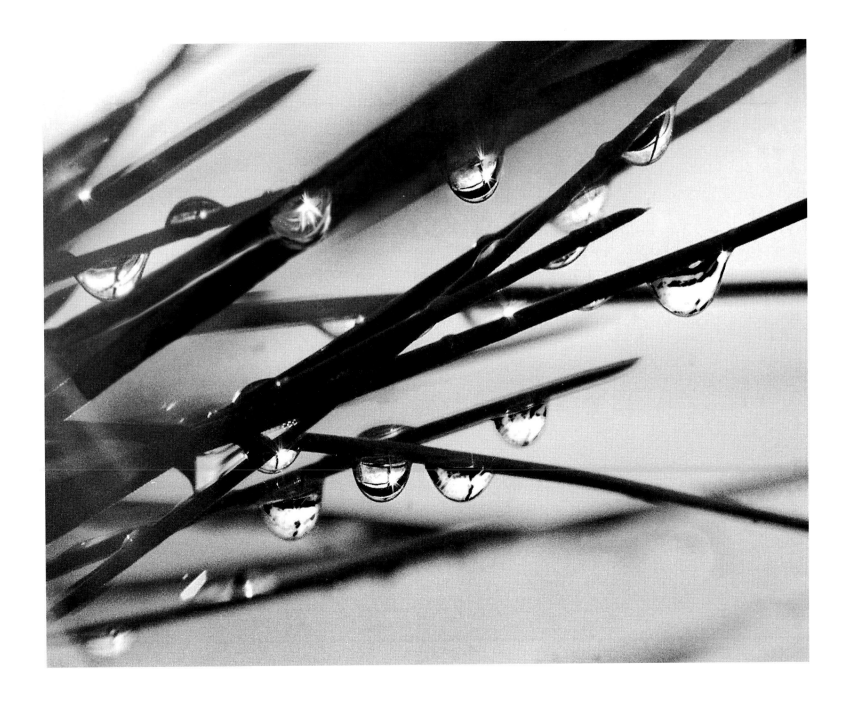

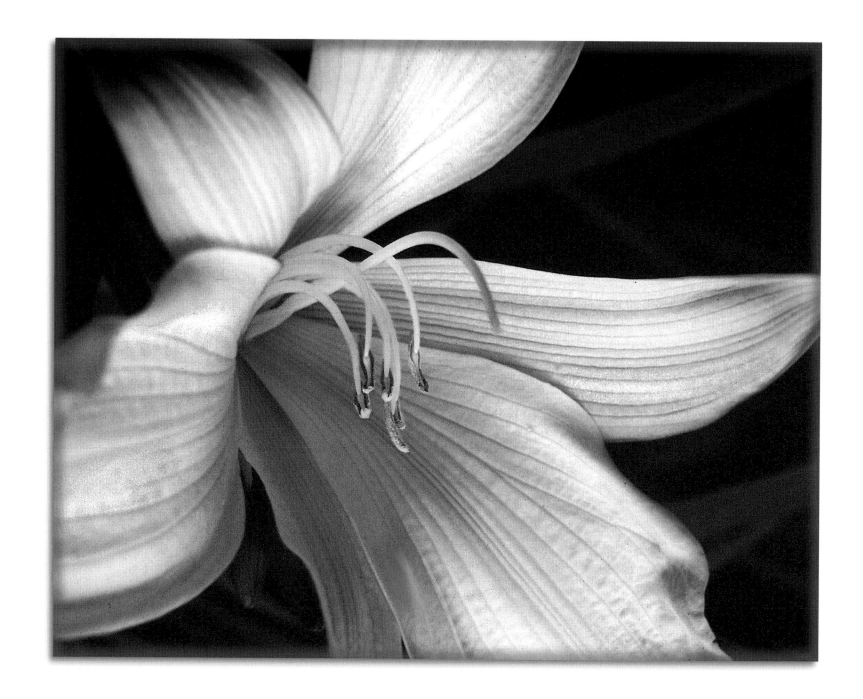

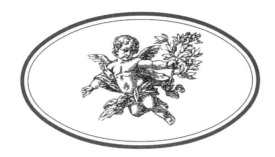

THE TOUGH QUESTIONS

"God enters by a private door into every individual"
— Ralph Waldo Emerson

I call Children's Hospital the Miracle House; and my name for it is rightly deserved. Miracles large and small happen there every day. I have witnessed many with my own eyes.

In contrast to the stark environment of an adult hospital, the colors on the walls of the Miracle House are bright and welcoming. But despite the beautiful and loving decor, to someone entering for the first time from the outside world, the place can feel daunting and disorienting, like visiting a foreign country.

Recently arrived families must cope with so many things all at once. They are attempting to make the most important decisions of their lives while learning an alien geography and adjusting to the unfamiliar medical culture and language of their newly adopted "country."

In the

depth of winter,

I finally learned

that within me

there lay

an invincible

summer.

— Albert Camus

A ward volunteer has the opportunity to be the bridge between these two worlds — a citizen from another country helping recently-arrived immigrants adjust to their new surroundings. The assignment can range from showing relatives how to navigate their way around the hospital, to making them feel more at home by bringing them a warm cup of tea, and sharing joys, fears, and heartfelt concerns.

Throughout the years I have seen families of all religious persuasions come through the hospital doors. The doctors, nurses, staff, and volunteers have respectfully bowed their heads while prayers have been uttered in Hebrew, Arabic, Hindi, Japanese, Spanish, and Russian.

You don't have to speak the language to understand one question all parents ask in disbelief, "Why?"

When our loved ones are ailing, questions arise from our souls to which the answers are perhaps known only to a power greater than human comprehension. Our processes for seeking peace are uniquely personal and entirely private. Yet, as a ward volunteer, I am in the midst of these private moments all of the time. I have had my own struggle finding peace in the face of overwhelming sorrow. During my first few years at the hospital, I often drove home crying almost uncontrollably. Eventually, I found the peace I was seeking. For me, the answer was in the thirteenth chapter of First Corinthians, "For now we see through a glass, darkly; but then face to face. Now I understand in part; but then I shall fully understand even as I am fully understood. And now abide faith, hope, love, these three; but the greatest of these is love."

This idea brings me comfort. It reminds me that no matter how much science advances, and how hard physicists may try to explain the mysteries of the unseen, they cannot see all there is to see, nor can I. There will always be mysteries that baffle the mind and open the heart.

Each of us grapples with soul-searching questions at some point in our lives. Religion comes into this book because these are actual stories and people in crisis turn to their faith. Families who are adjusting to the "foreign territory" of the Miracle House often gather strength through the religion of their heritage.

Over time, I have come to see religion as a container for faith. While the containers may vary in size and shape, the contents are universal. We all have the same essential qualities in common, ". . . faith, hope and love, but the greatest of these is love."

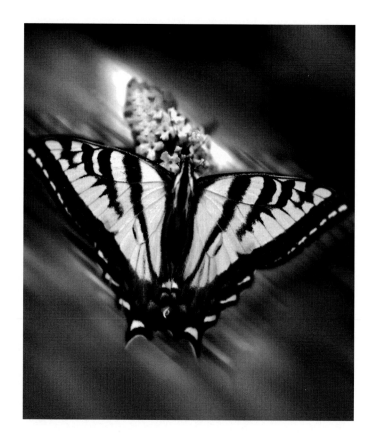

In India, heaven is believed to be a network of pearls. These pearls are arranged in a divine order of multiple reflections. If you look at one, you see all the others reflected in it. Similarly, many in the scientific community now realize that each particle of matter is not merely itself but involves every other particle. All are in some way intertwined, and everything we do affects the whole.

— An interpretation of a holographic view of reality, based upon a classic Buddhist sutra.

CHAPTER SIX = I'LL DO BETTER NEXT TIME

"First you have to go deep inside yourself to find your answers. You can tell you are getting the answer when your heart and belly get warmer. Courage is power from the heart. You feel like, 'This is pretty scary! But I have to do it sometime, so let's do it now!' And then you just look straight ahead and you make yourself do it. But be careful to be honest and kind."

— Lydia W. = 8 years old

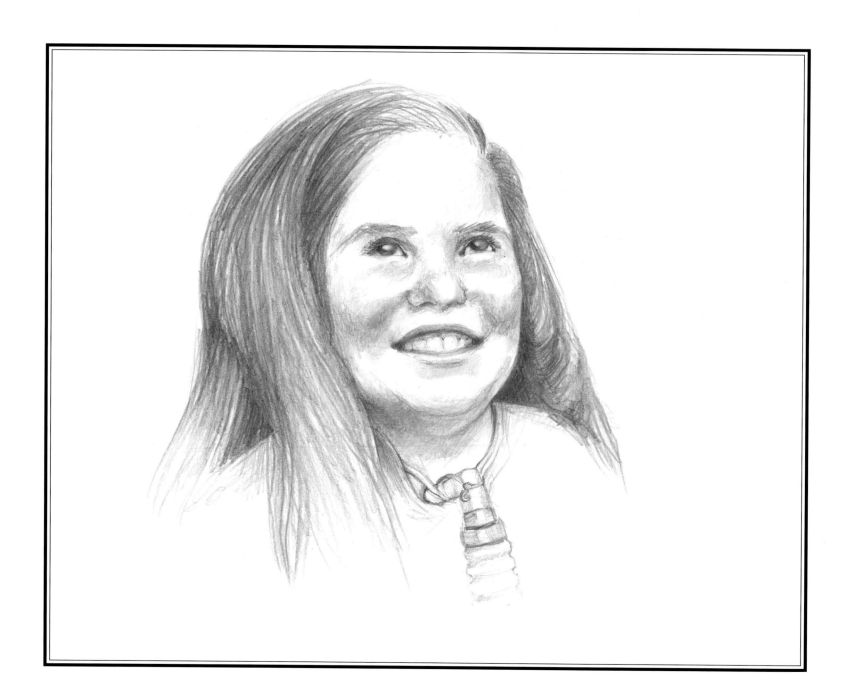

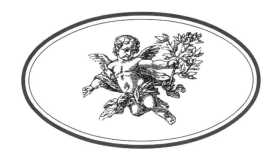

I'LL DO BETTER NEXT TIME

"Turn your face to the sun and the shadows will fall behind you."

— Maori Proverb

I encountered my first young shooting victim in the intensive care unit. Green numbers, electronic beeps, and wavy lines offered comforting assurance to concerned staff and family. Just moments earlier this ten-year-old girl accompanied a family member to a target range where the breech of a gun had exploded. A wayward piece of steel instantly severed her spinal cord very close to her brain stem. One moment she was playing happily, the next moment she could no longer breathe, move, or communicate. She was terrified.

Unable to move anything but her head and tongue, she was adjusting to a tracheotomy, twenty-four-hour care and the unnatural sound of the ventilator — her new constant companion. Her prognosis was bleak.

I gently introduced myself to this severely injured child. At first she seemed lost in a bundle of pink coverlet, then her eyes suddenly locked onto mine with an unwavering sense of determination. This first meeting began an enduring relationship with a dynamic spirit whose years in the Miracle House influenced hundreds of lives, especially my own.

I saw her every week for more than a decade. Her pre-teen years were filled with Girl Scout activities. She sold cookies from a gurney up and down the long corridors. Without the use of her limbs, her animated selling techniques were restricted to her sparkling blue eyes and bright smile. Every year, she raised hundreds of dollars for her troop.

I looked forward to our weekly visits and always followed her explicit instructions. She was the dictator, and I was the foot soldier closely adhering to her artistic commands. I learned the names of all her colorful goldfish, provided physical assistance when she was rug hooking by mouth, and maintained her meticulous bonsai collection. She was bold, frank, and intense. One day she snapped at me while I was trimming her bonsai tree.

"You almost ruined it! You cut it too short!" she admonished. "I don't like you tonight! Go home!" I received these marching orders on more than one occasion and always replied with a grin. Then, looking back over my shoulder, I gave her that wink that she knew so well and added with a lilt in my voice, "Okay, but I'll be back next week!"

Early in our relationship we decided on nicknames. Hers was "Blue Eyes." A most beautiful shade of blue, her eyes could change abruptly depending on her mood or frame of mind. Pain, fear, and determination had their own intensity, yet these windows to her soul took on a particular clarity when she spoke about her enduring faith. My nickname was "Grasshopper" for my animated antics and rapidly shifting ideas for entertainment over the many bleak hours.

At the age of twelve she began to paint by mouth. One surprising day she insisted that her very first effort be entered in the local county fair. "Why are you going to so much trouble?" I asked.

"To see how much it will sell for!" she replied happily.

The following week her enthusiastic greeting nearly bowled me over. Her expression was clear and strong in spite of her tracheotomy. "Grasshopper! Grasshopper! They sold my painting!"

"And what did they give you for it?"

"A piece of paper over there, on the shelf!" It was a check, of course, made out to the young artist. "How do we turn it into money?" she asked impatiently.

"You'll have to endorse it." Her blue eyes tunneled into mine as she awaited further instructions. I placed a thick-barreled pen into her mouth. "Now, write your name."

"Okay," she said eagerly. Her face was flushed from the endorsement effort. "Now, where is my money?" I reached into my change pocket and reluctantly cashed her check, carefully laying a total of sixty cents on her bed.

She stared at the coins in disbelief. All was silent except the sound of her ventilator. After a long pause she simply said, ". . . I'll do better next time." I was staggered by this response. She had spent so many hours with a brush in her mouth dreaming of this day, this very moment, and now here it was.

In an instant she allowed all the feelings to wash over her as she reframed the situation in her mind. Rather than sinking into a sense of defeat, she saw the incident as a small victory — smaller than she had hoped — but a victory just the same. "Blue Eyes" continued to develop her artistic talent with hours and hours of practice. Before long, her mastery over her craft rivaled that of many published artists twice her age who were painting with their hands.

At the age of fifteen she completed two Christmas cards. One painting contained three figures: Joseph, Mary, and the donkey. The other design included small, intricate trees in the landscape. Her detailed technique was astounding, and her artwork was soon published. The hospital sold forty-five thousand of these cards. Katie donated the proceeds to the Uncompensated Care Fund for other hospitalized children.

My mind once again revisited the moment when I reluctantly placed only sixty cents on her bedside and wondered, "What if this had happened to me?" I think I would have been deeply disappointed and humiliated.

What would *I* have said? I believe my response would have been *No more.*
I give up! When defeating thoughts such as these come to mind now, I find myself instantly recalling Katie's encouraging words, "I'll do better next time."

As the years passed, our weekly chats developed a familiar comfort about them. She reviewed her hospital activities of the previous seven days, and I shared my daily challenges in the marketplace. One quiet evening in her fourteenth year I reflected on our relationship, "Blue Eyes, you have been in that bed for over three years. I'd be surprised if you were not bitter over the accident that has left you like this."

"Oh, no," she quickly replied, "God chose me to have this experience, and I would have been very disappointed had He chosen anyone else!"

With her sixteenth birthday just weeks away, she decided on a very special place to celebrate. Confined to her bed in a tiny room day after day, she wanted to make the most of this rare outing. She chose to be six hundred feet in the air at the Seattle Space Needle where the restaurant revolves once every hour. There she would be, sitting on top of the world, watching the shimmering water of the Puget Sound as it wove its way through immense forests and disappeared into the distant mountain ranges below.

Would she consider voice invitations? Of course not. Every single invitation was mouth written. Family members, close friends, and Mr. and Mrs. Grasshopper all received individual labors of love enclosed in a personally inscribed envelope.

When the special day finally arrived, Blue Eyes was beaming in her new white floor-length gown. The outpouring of love for her guests was reflected by their enduring love for her. I pondered about a gift and finally settled on a special letter which I read aloud:

Dear Sweet Sixteen,

What visions and feelings come to mind when those two words relate to my dear friend Katie! It has been almost six years now since we first met. What changes you have brought to your life.

From a bundle of fear huddled beneath a pink coverlet you have become a beautiful, mature young lady, self-confident, self-reliant, and filled to overflowing with a vibrant spirit. The little girl things of yesterday have been put away. The Girl Scout cookies, merit badges, and Raggedy Ann dolls are all gone now. Earrings, perfumes, lipsticks, and intellectual treatises galore adorn your shelves.

With your artistic talents honed to a professional stature, your plans for living and working in the real world have taken on a deeper meaning. Yet, throughout this transformation some things haven't changed and, God willing, never will. Your warm smile, the dancing lights in your lovely eyes, and the strength of your steel-strong spirit meld all of your character traits — honesty, compassion, and sensitivity to name but a few.

All of these things are cemented together with an abiding, deep-seated faith.

Throughout the years I have found you ministering to me in ways beyond description. May your next years yield everything your sixteen-year-old heart might wish for — peace, contentment, and finally, fulfillment of those most precious dreams of all, those you keep hidden from everyone but God.

You are precious and priceless. Happy Birthday!

Love, Grasshopper

As she grew older she dreamed of having her own home. She longed to be free from the constraints of hospital life with its strict adherence to daily planned activities. We pored over the real estate ads and sales brochures together. She sketched detailed plans for every room of her dream house. The designs included space for her involved medical equipment, sleeping quarters for her twenty-four-hour care givers, and all the necessities her condition demanded.

We were planning her future when a strange question spontaneously sprang out, "Katie, I'm tired of seeing you in that bed, week after week, month after month.

When are you going to get up and walk?" I was stunned by my own words, yet she responded without hesitation.

"I'm going to get up one of these evenings and walk down that corridor. There will be three of us," she continued. "I'll be in the middle, you'll be on one side, and Jesus will be on the other."

Her faith, strong from the beginning, was further refined as she read the Bible from cover to cover three times, with the aid of a page turner. She thoroughly enjoyed chiding me as she posed Biblical questions to which I pleaded ignorance. All the while she burnished my own faith as well as that of many others.

It was a sunny spring morning when the call came. I was just about to be introduced for a speaking engagement. My wife, Helen, was on the phone. "The hospital just called. Blue Eyes passed away moments ago."

My surroundings became a complete blur. I felt my heart breaking in two. As I closed my eyes and wept, a clear image appeared in my mind. I could see her finally walking down the hallway as promised. . .

"There will be three of us . . . "

My dear Katie, thank you for being my life teacher. I promised myself I would document your guidance and share it with others, and now here it is.

Can you imagine how different our world would be if each of us heard your simple words within our own minds every time we were indulging in a sense of failure?

" . . . I'll do better next time."

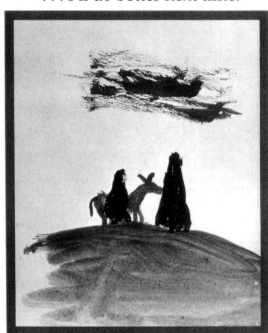

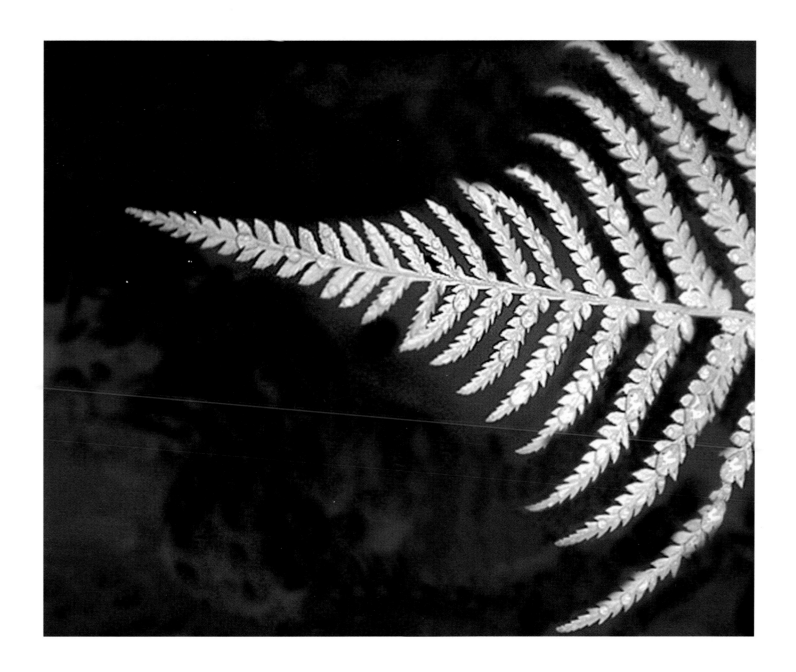

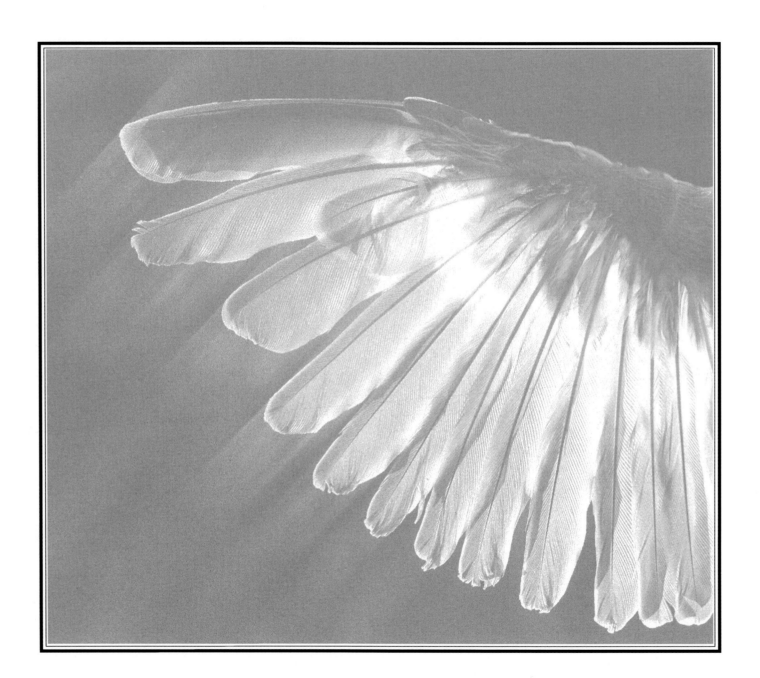

CHAPTER SEVEN - SO BE IT

"My dad says everyday is a good day, even if it is a bad day. If you complain to him he always says, 'This is a beautiful day and if you don't enjoy it, it's your own darn fault!' He is usually right, even when he is wrong for awhile, then he is right again by bedtime."
— Roger M. - 10 years old.

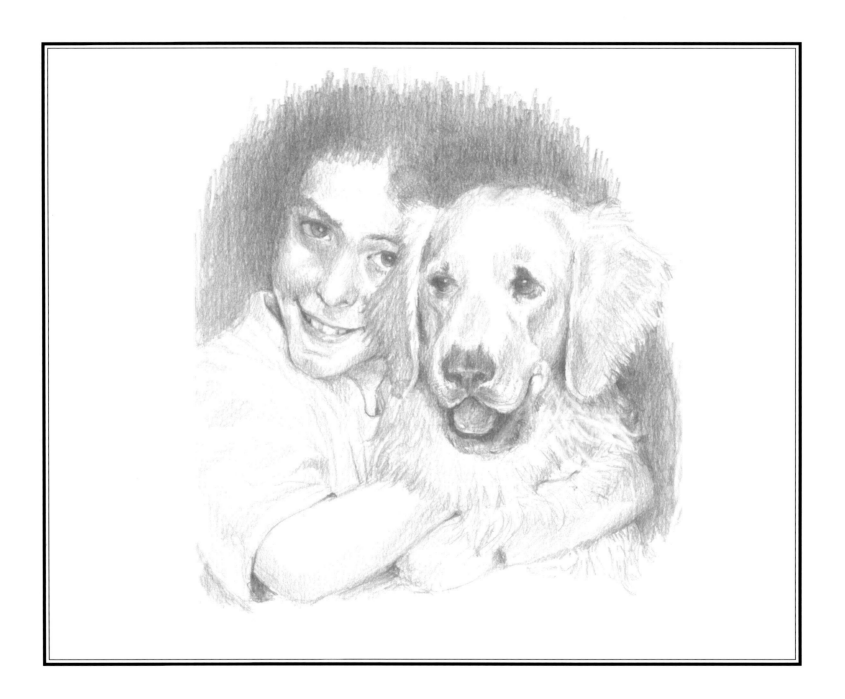

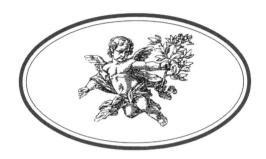

SO BE IT

"Be kind, for everyone you meet
may be fighting a harder battle." — Plato

It was one of those magic Northwest afternoons. The sky was cloud-less. A soft wind came out of the north. The combined fragrance of cedar trees and newly mown turf mingled in the air. I walked off the green toward the clubhouse to change my shoes in preparation for the evening's silent auction and dinner. It would be another charitable event, with the proceeds donated to hospitalized children.

We met just before being seated at the same table. The ten-year-old boy's soft brown eyes welcomed me into his soul as he introduced himself. Thus, the young teacher and the seasoned car salesman began a relationship that was destined to change both of their lives.

Colt was his name, and cancer was his enemy. The enemy first made its presence known in the young boy's right leg. When it came time to decide whether or not to amputate, he accepted his fate with grace and conviction. Without a trace of resignation his reply was, "Let's get on with it." The procedure was soon history, and the healing began. He did not dwell on the things that he could not change. Demonstrating the essence of grace, time and time again he seemed to say, "So be it." This attitude became an profound aspect of my own approach to life.

Over the years I was honored to accompany this bright young hero to his innumerable operations. Before entering the operating room each time, I would kiss him on the forehead and tell him how proud I was of him. Two stem cell transplants, total body radiation, and multiple episodes of chemotherapy gave us the opportunity to enrich our friendship.

As time passed I offered hand-holding, voiced my encouragement, and attempted to shoulder a portion of the load this young man carried with such grace and determination. His greatest support came from his blessed mother, Pattie, who was always there, night and day, throughout his many recoveries. She was the backbone of his enduring stand for life.

Among our many shared experiences over the years, one clearly stands out. Colt was in the hospital and very ill after repeated chemotherapy treatments. He was truly in critical condition. I entered the room cautiously. Mom was standing in the corner. I couldn't help but blurt out, "Colt, you look awful! Pattie, what's his platelet count?" (Normally it should have been 375,000 to 500,000.)

"It's down to 6000," Pattie replied with resignation in her voice.

"Colt, that's terrible! I'll tell you what I'm going to do. I'm going to give you half of mine. I have four extra-special ones, and you're going to get two of them!" Colt's expression hardly changed. He was sucking shaved ice to ease the pain of the huge sores in his mouth and throat.

Patty laughed softly and said, "Now what are you up to?"

"Well, I'm not certain, but I'll be back tomorrow with the platelets."

I stood in the parking lot, closed my eyes for a moment and asked, "Dear God, you heard the promise I just made. What now?"

The image came quickly. I saw the Goodwill Store clearly in my mind. I parked the car, went through the front entrance, and listened for intuitive guidance. I felt the urge to turn left through a doorway, then left again. I found myself in a small room displaying bric-a-brac of every description.

In the middle was a glass case filled with smaller items. On the second shelf, in the corner, there they were! Four small plates, three inches in diameter, with a Chinese character in the center. Each one was bright red. Four tiny plates. *Platelets!* "Thank you God," I whispered aloud. With the four tissue-wrapped treasures in my pocket I waited impatiently for the next day.

My anticipation continued to mount as I approached his room. I had to muster all of my self-control to avoid bursting through the door. "Colt, before I give you half of my platelets, I want you to answer a couple of questions. First, what is a small eagle called?" In no mood for a quiz, Colt shook his head in silence.

"An eaglet, Colt...." I continued, "How about a small pig...?" Again, there was no response. "A piglet, Colt... Try *harder*...! A small plate...?"
Colt thought for moment and then muttered weakly, "A platelet?"

"Right, and here they are!" I carefully unwrapped two of the platelets and placed them in his pale, damp hands. A smile returned to his face as he began enjoying the whole charade. Pattie's laughter tumbled into the room as the door closed behind me.

The next day his platelet count had increased remarkably. Had I witnessed a miracle? I had no idea why I promised to bring him exactly four "platelets." Nor did I have any idea how I would find them or what the ancient Chinese characters inscribed upon them meant. A shudder rippled through me when I recently learned the translation for the repeated message each one carried, "Longevity . . . *Longevity* . . . ."

Several years have passed. Colt is now seventeen. He is back in school, drives his own car, plays golf, and meets every new challenge with courage, determination, and a wonderful smile.

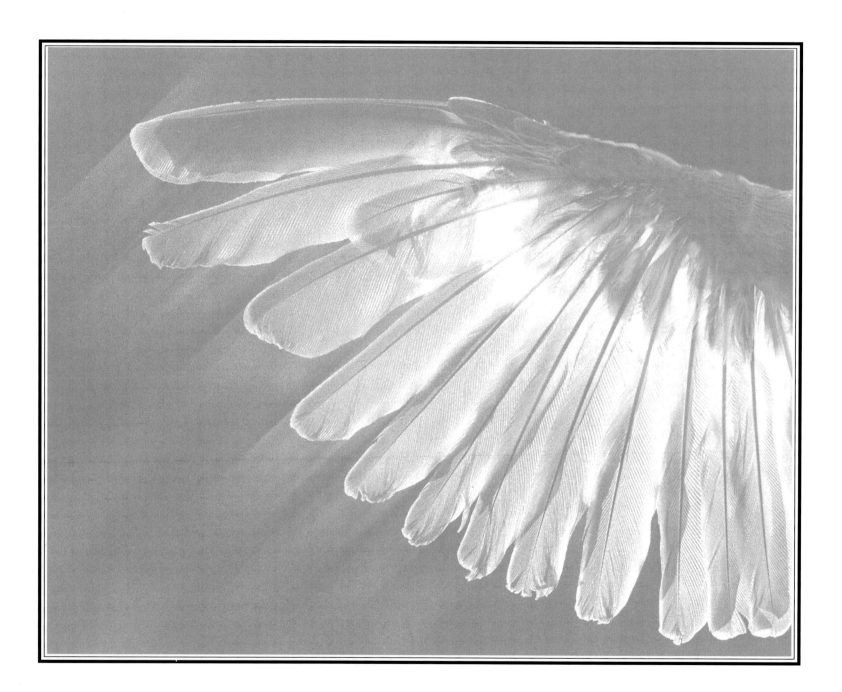

CHAPTER EIGHT ~ UNCOMMON STRENGTH

"If you see someone in a wheelchair or walking with a cane, try and help them open the door because it is hard to do. Don't worry about embarrassing them because they would be happy to know that you cared about them. It doesn't matter how you look on the outside, like if some one has a scar from being in a fire. A person might look different from everyone else on the outside, but on the inside they could be just as good as everyone else or even better!"

— Samantha S. ~ 16 years old.

"Give the world

the best

you have to give

and you may get hurt.

Give the world your best

anyway...

People are unreasonable,

illogical,

and self-centered.

Love them

anyway..."

—Mother Teresa

When he came to the Miracle House, Billy's fingers looked like tapered candles. His strong will sustained him through painful multiple surgeries, skin grafts and arduous treatments. The tender child behind the burn mask innocently frightened his young contemporaries merely by looking in their direction.

He endured the challenges of chronic pain, extended hospitalization, and rejection by his peers. Only a steel-clad inner strength could withstand such tremendous trials.

Billy and I became friends during my weekly rounds at the Hospital. His tenacity astounded me.

Despite the skillful efforts of plastic surgeons, his former appearance could not be restored. Nevertheless, he continued to heal and get stronger in every respect. Finally, he was well enough to leave the Miracle House.

Billy soon learned that fire had changed more than his outward appearance. It also changed the troubles he faced in life. At school, he was the subject of merciless teasing. Once again, he relied on his strong will. He turned his focus to his school-work and continued to heal his body.

In the spring of that same year, the Anti-Defamation League was having a celebration dinner downtown. They asked Helen and me if we wanted to invite one of my "kids" to the dinner. Even though he was only six years old, I asked Billy to join us. He certainly knew the pain of personal attack and had endured it with courageous patience. He had my absolute respect and admiration. I could not imagine a more appropriate guest.

At the end of the dinner, following an evening focused on diversity, equality and human rights, Billy was offered the chance to speak. He willingly consented. Mindful of his healing process, I carefully lifted him up onto the podium and adjusted the microphone. He suddenly found himself to be taller than everyone else in the room. It occurred to me that after everything he had been through, this small boy did indeed stand taller than the rest of us.

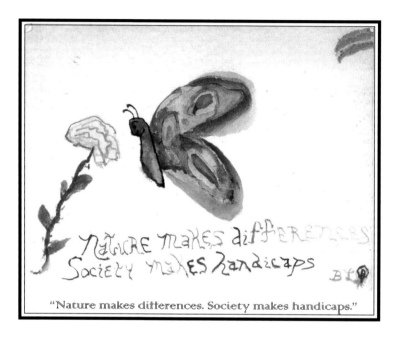

"Nature makes differences. Society makes handicaps."

I have had a lot of experience with kids being mean to me. When you are being teased it feels like your heart could explode. It is the worst feeling in the world. You have to get away for awhile. You have to remember that their hearts are not strong enough to be kind. I can be stronger than that. They want to act cool because they are so worried about how they look to other people. They try to make other people look bad, so they can look good. But it doesn't make them look good. Faces look ugly when they are being mean. I started feeling sorry for them because they felt the need to tease me."

— Megan S. - 11 years old

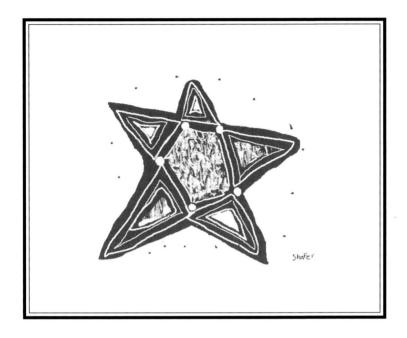

"It is hard to be kind to someone who hurts you. It takes awhile, but you can forgive them. It feels really good because the anger isn't inside of you anymore. It wasn't your anger anyway." Megan S. – 11 years old

"If you are having a hard time just keep saying, "You can do it. Never give up!" You can say that to yourself and it really helps. And you can talk to your good friend. A good friend is someone who makes you feel better."

— Shafer S. – 7 years old

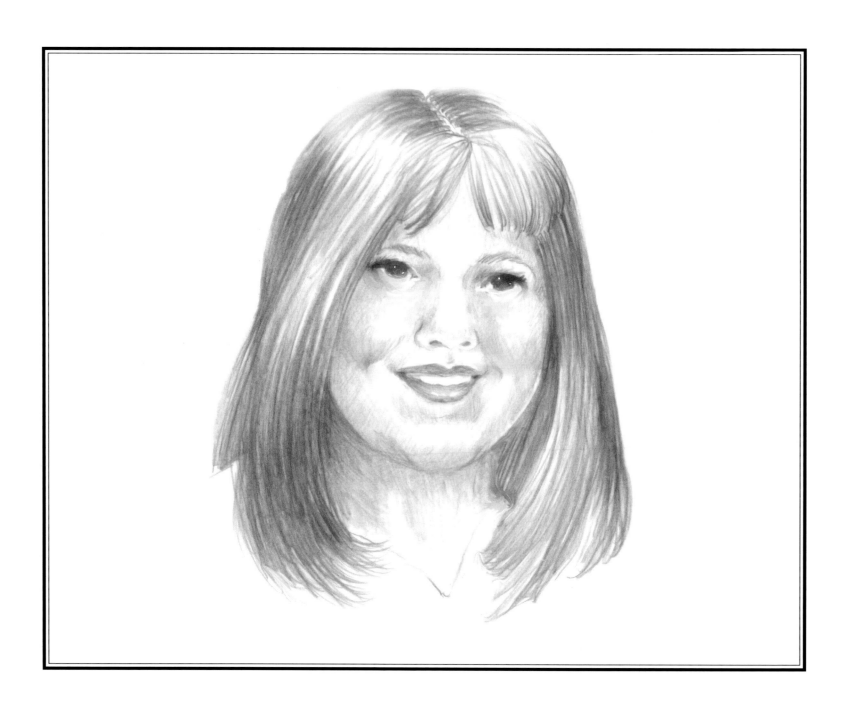

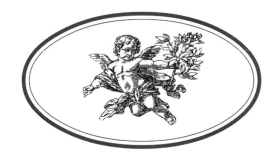

LEARNING TO LISTEN

"We never listen when we are eager to speak."

— Francois, Duc de la Rochefoucauld

Helen's caution every time I venture onto a freeway is consistent and caring, "Stay awake and don't drive too close!"

"All right," I assured her, "I'll call you when I get there and again when I arrive back at the dealership." My destination this time was Aberdeen, Washington, a small town primarily dependent upon logging and fishing. I had been invited to share the *third eight* with the high school student body. While I was looking forward to my time with the youth, I was not looking forward to the two-and-a-half hour drive in heavy traffic.

Standing backstage I could see the students pouring into the large auditorium. These colorful young men and women reminded me of birds in an open field.

"Appreciation
is a wonderful
thing;
it makes what is
excellent
in others
belong to us
as well."

—Voltaire

They were chirping with raucous laughter in flurries of animated activity. The teenage fluttering eventually subsided and all eyes settled on me. In the deepening silence, my desire to teach the *third eight* mounted. I was determined to have this moment count. I wanted to change the way these young people viewed their lives here on earth.

Midway through the presentation a young girl in the front row caught my eye. I walked up to her and asked her name. "Naomi," she answered shyly.

"Naomi, are you aware that there's never been another young woman exactly like you? No matter how many times this earth has revolved on its axis, or made its full journey around the sun, no other Naomi has lived your life or had your thoughts. Over the last one million years and throughout the entire history of the world, there has never been, nor will there ever be, another Naomi with your character, your courage, and your dreams for the future. How are you going to use your entirely unique gifts?"

I could almost hear the thoughts whizzing through her mind. Her eyes widened. Then a knowing smile settled on her face. I had no idea what she was thinking, but it was clear that she was sorting things out.

Turning to a young man seated near her I asked, "And your name please?" He cast his eyes to the floor and self-consciously answered, "Jacob."

"Did you know that you can make a difference in this world, Jacob? Well, you can. What part of the world are *you* going to change?"

I looked back at the audience, "Each one of us in this room here today can and will have an influence on the world. We can't know how long we will live. Some of us will live to old age and others will not. The exact number of our days remains a mystery. The question is, what will you do with your unique God-given talents? When your life has ended, will you have left anything behind besides your social security number?

"How will you use this day, this week, this glorious life of yours?"

Each time I speak with young people the experience is different, and yet somehow the same. As the lights dim, they see a businessman step onto the stage with a microphone clipped to his collar. The kids make themselves comfortable and settle in for the lecture. Soon the scene changes. I am down among the chairs with them, and the businessman becomes a surrogate grandfather who is lovingly asking more from them than they ask of themselves.

As the students left the darkened hall, I wondered how many of them were still waiting for their lives to begin and how many actually knew that their lives mattered now? While collecting my things backstage, I noticed a young lady standing nearby. Her eyes were beginning to brim with tears. She looked at me steadily and spoke six words I will never forget. "I want to be like you."

Ill-prepared for such a comment, I fumbled for my handkerchief and slowed the flow of tears trailing down her cheeks. "What's your name?" I asked.

"April," she replied.

"How old are you?"

"Sixteen."

"And you want to be like me?"

She clutched my handkerchief and quietly nodded her head.

I frantically searched for the proper response but my mind just kept telling me, "I don't know what to say. What should I say?" I took a breath, settled into a comfortable silence and waited for my heart to speak. After a while the words came. "April, you have been like me since the day you were born. You feel the way you do because you recognize yourself in me."

In my mind's eye I can still clearly see her walking up the long aisle leading out of the auditorium and back to her classroom. As she vanished from sight I knew she would never be far from my heart.

A soft rain clouded the afternoon sky. The windshield wipers drummed a slow rhythm keeping pace with the questions rolling through my mind. I wondered how many of these young people would begin to consciously contribute their *third eight*? How many *third eight* hours of contribution walked out of that room today? If only ten of them gave away a small piece of their time each week for the rest of their lives, what would be the potential there? The *third eight* squared? Cubed? And what was young April's gift to me?

I believe her gift was the way she taught me how to listen. Young people are expected to listen to adults but more importantly, we must change the way we listen to them. April taught me to surrender my need to know the answers and listen from the vulnerable place of not knowing. When we quiet our minds, our hearts open on their own. It is in this place that we can listen for these young souls' innermost thoughts, viewpoints and concerns about life.

I pulled the car into the garage. Helen met me at the door and asked how it went. I hung my overcoat in the closet and began recounting the events of the day. When I came to the part about April, I looked into Helen's eyes and suddenly became aware of how busy my mind had been. I stopped and just listened to her, even though she wasn't saying anything. Helen's eyes were steady and familiar. She tilted her head slightly, and I saw my beautiful bride of sixty years. Overwhelmed with appreciation, I pulled her into my arms and whispered, "I love you."

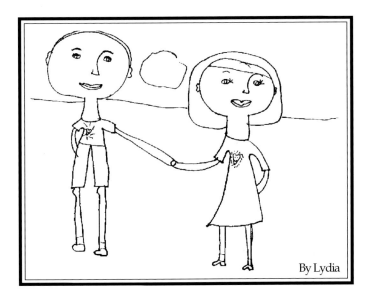

By Lydia

"A good friend is someone who encourages you and makes you laugh and makes you feel better when you are sad."

CHAPTER TEN - IF I BE RELAXED AND FREE

"I love to play sports! Any game, anytime.

You name it, and I am there! I love the snow too.

If it is snowing, you'll know I'm happy."

— Nathan H. - 13 years old

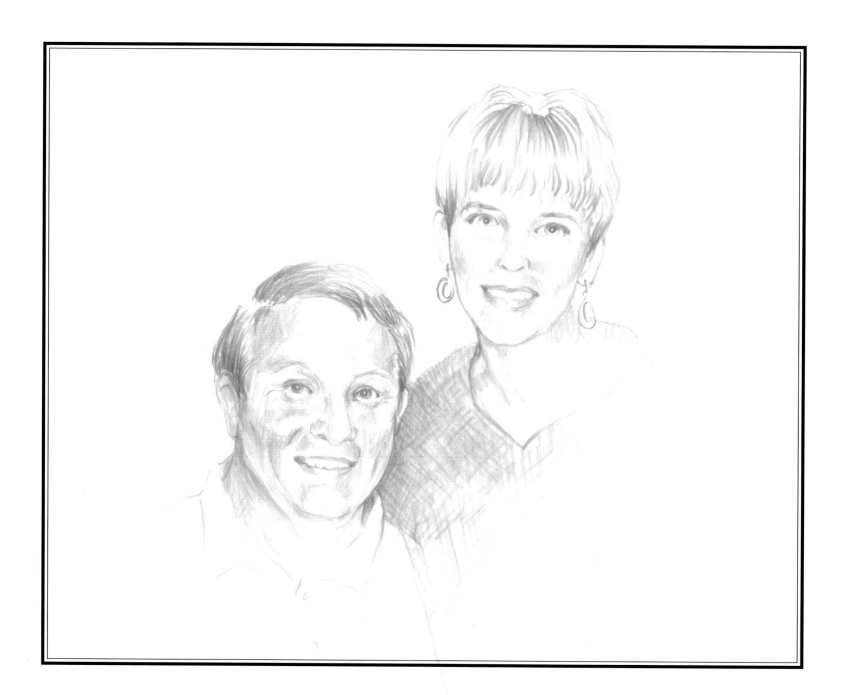

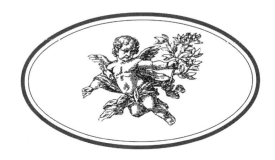

IF I BE RELAXED AND FREE

"I have learned from experience that the greater part of our happiness or misery depends on our dispositions and not on our circumstances." — Martha Washington

Jeff Sykes had always wanted to play football. He loved the excitement of each action-filled moment: the intense focus on the game, the smell of the turf churning under his cleats, and the light-filled stadiums crowded with teachers, parents, families, and classmates cheering him on. By the time he reached high school he had achieved the physical and mental discipline necessary to make the team. He practiced daily from midsummer into fall. Every day after school and each Saturday were dedicated to practice, practice and more practice.

An October breeze carried the welcome scent of distant bonfires onto the field. After school, teenagers leaned against parked cars and gathered near the bleachers. The whistle blew. The huddle broke. The line tensed, and the ball was snapped.

Helmets clattered as the teammates piled onto one another. The ball carrier broke away and headed into the open field, only one player left between himself and the end zone. They put their heads down and ran full speed toward each other, like two rams unwilling to give up an inch of territory. They hit. Silence fell over the field, and the team froze in disbelief. One of their own lay motionless far too long.

Jeff was sixteen years old when we first met. I was making my rounds one Wednesday evening when I noticed a young man stretched out on a revolving bed. He was lying face down with just about two feet between his face and the floor. I stood outside his door and said, "Why do they have you in that contraption?" A strong voice answered from under the bed, "I broke my neck and smashed two vertebrae, C5 and C6."

"Why do you have to be face down?"

"They turn me on this thing like a rotisserie. Sometimes I get to look at the ceiling, sometimes the floor. Right now, it's the floor."

He seemed like such a fine young man. I found myself straining to see his face. "When I talk to people, I like to look into their eyes. Do you mind if I slide under your bed?" I took off my jacket, stretched out on the floor and scooched my way in.

There we were, nose to nose, no more than a few inches apart when Jeff whispered to me, "You've got a lot of nerve crawling under this bed in your three-piece suit!"

He told me the whole story: the hit he took during a team scrimmage, the ambulance arriving at the scene, and the two surgeries that followed. He was concerned about his mom and dad. "The doctors had to remove the bone fragments near my spine. They didn't know if I was going to make it through the surgery. This has been tough on my parents."

A pair of white shoes quickly trotted up to the bed. "What's going on here?" asked an authoritative voice.

With as much dignity as possible I answered, "I'm a ward volunteer just visiting with my new friend here."

"This is not the proper way to...Don't you know how we. . ." With each stammering attempt at correcting my behavior she sounded less and less official. "This is not the way we visit with. . .Well, I guess it's all right." She tried to contain herself as she made her way to the door, but I heard a giggle as she rounded the corner into the corridor.

What

you are,

the world is.

And

without your

transformation,

there

can be no

transformation

of the world.

— Krishnamurti

As the months passed, Jeff and I had a number of nose-to-nose conversations. My admiration for him grew each time we met. I asked him about his depth of concentration. How could he be so intently focused on his recovery and, at the same time, so consistently good-natured? He answered, "Most things I take on as a challenge. I see this as just another challenge in my life." These words hung in the air for a moment and then settled deeply in my heart.

Jeff had loved sports all of his life. He had been playing competitively since he was eleven years old. He was only sixteen at the time of the accident. His entire world revolved around his athletic abilities.

I tried to imagine losing my capacity to do the things I love most in the world. I wondered what my response might be.

Rather than giving up, Jeff immediately began to apply his dedication and talent to his current situation. He took on his devastating injury as "just one more challenge."

On more than one occasion the rehabilitation staff overheard Jeff coaching himself. Muttering under his breath he would say, "Never give up. Never give up. Always do your best. . . always your best." Whenever I reported on the progress of the other teens who were in rehab, Jeff was motivated to outperform himself.

Katie, a beautiful, lighthearted teenage girl, was recovering from a similar injury. On an outing one summer afternoon she had dived headlong into the shallows of a lake and broken her neck.

Although the circumstances of their accidents were different, I would tell Katie how well Jeff was doing, and she would compete against him. I would tell Jeff how well Katie was doing and his macho streak would flare up. I can still hear him saying, "No girl is going to be stronger than me!"

Throughout their recovery, I shared a special poem my mother had sent me during World War II. I had kept it posted near my bunk and committed it to memory:

I am the place where God shines through.
He and I are one not two.
I will not fear, nor fret, nor plan.
My place is where and as I am.
And if I be relaxed and free,
He will carry out His plan through me.

The line, "My place is where and as I am," can be the most difficult to grapple with when you are in the midst of a war as I was, or in the midst of a recovery as Jeff and Katie were. Yet it is precisely in those moments that accepting our circumstances opens the way to freedom.

Jeff continued to improve and eventually graduated from rehabilitation. The trophies he took with him were not the typical shiny towers of marble and gold. They were the personal victories of self-sufficiency, resilience, and independence. We said our good-byes and wished one another well. He rolled down the hall in one direction, opening the way to his new life, and I strolled down the hall in the other direction, opening the door to a new teacher.

One evening, more than twenty years later, I was continuing my rounds and visiting a patient when I heard a loud banging on the door behind me. I opened the door and saw a familiar looking man clad in a blue Hospital Volunteer coat.

He scooted his wheelchair in a bit closer and asked, "Are you Phil Smart?"

"Yes, I am," I nodded.

"Do you remember me?"

I studied the face of this man in his mid-thirties and said, "Let me think for a moment." The eyes. I knew those blue eyes. It couldn't be!

Before I could answer he said, "I'm Jeff Sykes!" I thought to myself, "How many years has it been? You are so grown up!" He must have read my face, because he laughed out loud. Then, with every muscle in his shoulders, he held out his arms. I reached out mine, and we embraced right there in the hallway.

"Phil, today I volunteer here at the hospital. Once a week, I'm on the hematology and oncology floor. I have so much to tell you!" he said. "I'm married now. I have a wonderful wife named Beverly, and I work as a database administrator with Boeing."

We met in the hospital cafeteria following our rounds and had a great time catching up. Jeff affectionately called his oncology assignment his "cancer kids" as he recounted the events leading to our reunion.

"I was late for my usual rounds with my cancer kids today because of a board meeting at Boeing. As I was signing in on the volunteer sheet I saw your name above mine. I couldn't believe it! I said, 'Is that Phil Smart, Senior? Is he still here after all these years?' They told me where to find you, and I was up there in no time flat."

"What brought you back to the Miracle House, Jeff?"

"So many things. . . I remembered how encouraging you were to me. I remembered how much better I performed when I had people cheering me on, so I became the one on the sidelines cheering others on. The way I see it, I am still on the team. I just have a different position now." As he was speaking, I thought back to that teenage boy, years ago, lying with his face down toward the floor and realized how much he had helped me see about myself. "This is just another challenge….Never give up….Cheer on the players and they will always perform better."

Jeff Sykes has been volunteering with his "cancer kids" for thirteen years now. He says they are his teachers. How well I understand! Jeff and I speak often. Every time he calls the dealership and gets my voice mail, he never leaves his name or number. Nevertheless, I always know it is Jeff.

His message? With his macho flair still shining through, he says, "I am the place where God shines through. He and I are one, not two. I will not fear, nor fret, nor plan. My place is where and as I am. And if I be relaxed and free, He will carry out his plan through me."

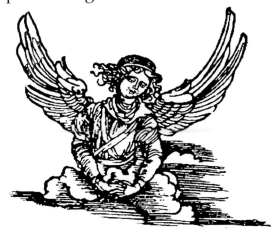

"To help the
young soul
redeem defeat
by new thought
and firm action,
this,
though not easy,
is the work of
divine man."

—Ralph Waldo Emerson

CHAPTER ELEVEN - PRESCRIPTION FOR PAIN

"I don't think you can choose a best friend.
But you can have lots of good friends. The
best way to get a friend is by kindness."

— Zachary S. - 11 years old

"If I could
reach up and hold
a star
for every time you've
made me smile,
the entire
evening sky
would be in the
palm of my hand."

— An Irish Saying

I checked in at the volunteer desk and was given a new assignment. "Tommy Hill, third floor, room 301."

He greeted me with a smile as wide as the bed. I could have fallen into that grin and been lost for a week. He was a strong, welcoming light, one that shone so brightly that the surroundings seemed to disappear. Yet, once my eyes adjusted, I noticed the maze of tubes connecting his body to a myriad of buzzing machinery.

The young Dr. Hill was good for my health. After a long day at the dealership, I could feel his loving eyes pouring into my soul. One memorable evening, as I appeared in the doorway, he turned and said, "Here comes that angel from Heaven." Can you imagine a car dealer being called an angel? I was certainly surprised!

He was small for his years and didn't seem to grow. I never saw him vertical, always in bed, in a chair, or on a gurney. He loved it when I read his favorite stories aloud. Our friendship deepened as we explored the world together through the pages of many dog-eared books. At night, he didn't like me to leave before he was asleep. I would always wait until his long dark lashes slowed their rhythm and closed completely before I tiptoed to the door. More often than not, he caught me. "Where are you going?"

"I'm going home now."

"But I'm not asleep yet!" And I would read another story.

It was Christmas Day of that same year when I entered his room clad in the Red Suit. Tommy was speaking to his grandfather on the telephone. Upon my arrival, he instantly interrupted the conversation, "Grandpa, the real Santa Claus is here! Talk to him!" I took the receiver in my gloved hand and introduced myself to Grandpa. Please keep in mind that while wearing the trappings of a legend, one becomes a bit bolder.

In a jovial spirit I said, "Hello, Gramps!"

A reserved voice responded at the other end of the line, "Yes, hello. How is my grandson Tommy?"

everyone he touched how to gain peace in the face of adversity. A letter I received shortly afterwards serves as a constant reminder of his gift.

Dear Mr. Smart,

I was so moved when you spoke with Thomas Hill on his deathbed. We all sat in the darkness, sad with our helplessness in not being able to save Thomas's life. The family and several staff members encircled his bed in silence until you said, "Please forgive me while I talk with my teacher here." You walked closer to Thomas and I will never forget the way you spoke to him:

"My dear young friend, I'm not sure I told you often enough how much you have taught me. You have been one of my finest teachers. You handled pain and fear so well. I love you and I will miss you greatly." And then you kissed him good-bye on the forehead.

When you walk into a room to spend time with a child who is attached to monitors and tubes, you see a child, not a patient. You always laugh and play with the children. It is so profound to me because you always remind me who it is lying in that bed or sitting in that wheelchair.

I know you dress up every Christmas to play Santa but you can't fool me. I know who you are. You are Santa who dresses up to play Phil Smart and pretends to sell cars.

Much love,
Kathy Salmonson
(Third floor nurse)

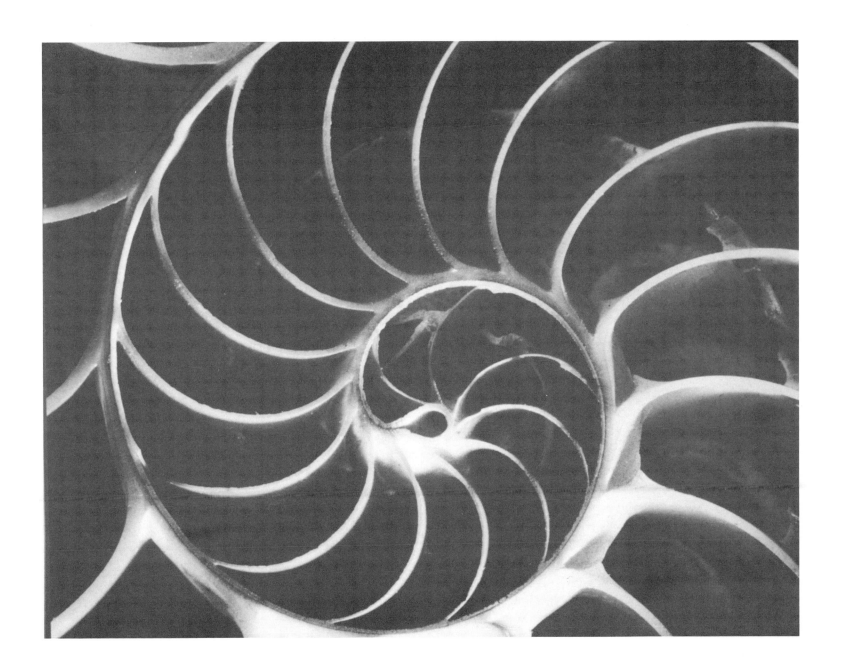

CHAPTER TWELVE ~ DON'T CALL ME DISABLED

"I have angels on my ceiling in my room. I painted them with my grandma. At night we sing about angels watching over me, over and over again. You can't get tired of that song when you are all snuggley with someone you love."

— Hannah P. ~ 7 seven years old.

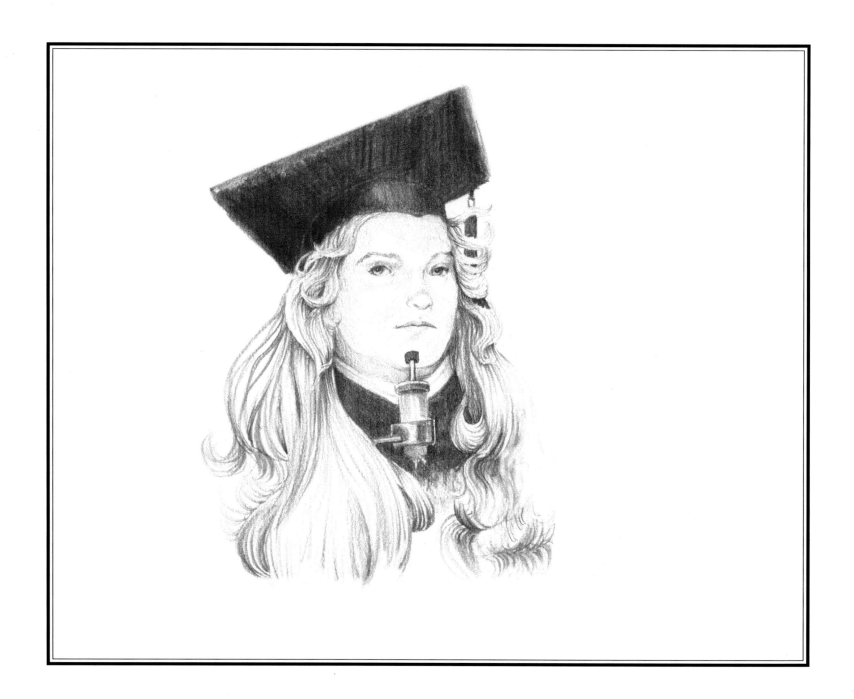

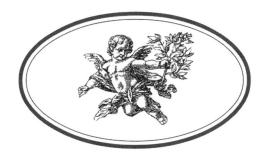

DON'T CALL ME DISABLED

"One can never consent to creep when one feels an impulse to soar."
— Helen Keller

It was a gorgeous day in Fairbanks, Alaska, when Bonnie's life-changing nightmare began. This beautiful nine-year-old child was sitting on her bed when a gun accident from the room next door changed her life in an instant. The shot pierced an adjoining wall, ricocheted off her bedspring, and tore through her neck. The bullet nicked her spinal cord, and the damage was irreversible.

It was instantly apparent to everyone at the Miracle House that Bonnie had been blessed with a remarkable spirit. Much like an athlete in training, she spent many hours, weeks, and months refining the skills she would need to win her independence. Throughout the course of her lengthy rehabilitation she learned to speak around the trachea tube that became the lifeline to her lungs.

> "If I am
>
> not
>
> for myself,
>
> then who
>
> am I for?
>
> If I am not for
>
> others,
>
> then who
>
> am I?"
>
> — Rabbi Hillel

Her level of mastery over the trach-tube equaled the hours of discipline and practice you and I would employ in order to become an opera singer. Normally when you are speaking, the air is going out of your lungs. With a trach-tube, you must speak while inhaling. Try it now and you will realize how difficult it is to merely communicate, let alone express your innermost feelings.

After months of physical therapy she returned to middle school in her new electric wheelchair. My admiration for her grew immeasurably as I thought about her entering the noisy school hallways and attempting to deal with both the physical and emotional barriers awaiting her arrival. At that age, all emotions become magnified.

The slightest difference in appearance can cause sleepless nights and embarrassment to the point of tears. While I was happy to see her go, I was concerned about her future. My concerns proved to be unfounded. Even at that tender age, Bonnie had an extraordinary ability to strive for her heart's desire. No obstacle was large enough to obscure her chosen path.

When she left the hospital so many years ago, I had no way of knowing that our friendship would endure forever. Bonnie faithfully wrote to me several times a year and we often spoke by phone. Helen and I were always thrilled to find Bonnie's notes in our mailbox. She always took the time to write the letters herself, holding a pen in her mouth. Each one was addressed to Santa.

Early one spring a mouth-addressed announcement arrived. "Bonnie Lynel Barber, graduate, Fairbanks High School." We were so proud of her! Our enthusiastic communications continued over the next four years until the day a formal announcement arrived from the University of Alaska at Fairbanks. Bonnie had earned her bachelor's degree.

College can be difficult under normal circumstances, and this young lady had met these challenges with the added difficulty of moving only her head and tongue. She often said to her peers, "Don't call me disabled! I have many abilities. If you must call me something, call me differently abled."

I can just imagine her racing around that campus like a thoroughbred amongst stable ponies. She was always encouraging others to run a good race while challenging everyone to meet her in the winner's circle.

By now she clearly recognized her unique talent for motivating others to reach beyond their self-imposed limitations. She was determined to obtain her master's degree in a profession that would allow her to further express her talents. Unfortunately, in spite of her high grade point average, she was rejected by one master's program after another. Within her field of study, it seemed as though there wasn't a university in the entire continent of North America that could accommodate her physical needs. Accepting her application meant accepting more than Bonnie alone. Her wheelchair, ventilator, and twenty-four-hour caregivers had to accompany her everywhere she went. Each day she hurried to her mailbox only to receive one rejection letter after another.

Bonnie could have conceded and obtained her degree through a correspondence program but she wanted to be among her peers, participate in classroom discussion and learn the information first hand. Undaunted, she relentlessly sought and found the perfect institution of higher learning to fulfill her goal. Several years later, she proudly sent the next announcement, "Bonnie Lynel

Barber, Master's Degree in Rehabilitation Counseling, University of Illinois."

One evening, Helen and I were enjoying a quiet dinner together when the telephone beckoned me away from the table. I considered letting it go and returning the call later, but even the telephone ring itself sounded insistent. "Santa, this is Bonnie."

"Where are you?"

"I'm at the Sea-Tac Airport. I want you to be at my motel tomorrow morning at 9 AM sharp!" That's the way she always is — to the point.

It was wonderful to see her again. I had barely taken my seat when she said, "Santa, I've made a decision about my future."

"And what might that be?"

"I'm going to get my Doctorate!"

"Bonnie, after all the struggles you've been through these many years, just what will you do with that degree?"

"Well, first of all I'll go back to the Miracle House, blow through those front doors in my electric wheelchair and then go up to the second floor, Rehab, where all of this began fifteen years ago."

"I'll be the one who counsels all of the patients who have suffered an injury like mine. Tell them to plan on my return — you know everyone there. You've been a part of that building for so many years, I figure you must have begun with the bricks!"

As you can imagine, it is difficult to talk Bonnie out of anything she sets her mind to. I felt that she was more than ready to apply her talents in the field of rehabilitation counseling and did not need any more schooling. She was a natural! She has a no-nonsense way of getting the most out of anyone with whom she shares her time. Whether it is an hour, a day, or just a brief moment, once you have been in her energetic presence you walk away shaking your head and wondering how you can do better in life. Over time she realized that her calling would not wait. School was in session, but not within the halls of another university.

Bonnie has specialized in rehabilitation counseling for eight years now. She carries a caseload of up to one hundred individuals challenged by alcoholism, drug addiction, and medical difficulties. Her clients know better than to give her any excuses. Her nature is hard-driving and her talent is clearly evident.

A thoroughbred in every respect, she challenges others to continually raise the bar and jump higher hurdles.

She is a true model of her degree, a Master.

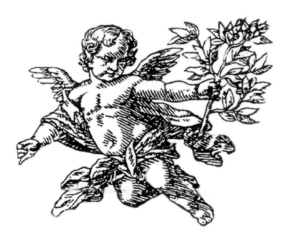

"There are only two ways to live your life. One is as though nothing is a miracle. The other is as though everything is a miracle."

— Albert Einstein

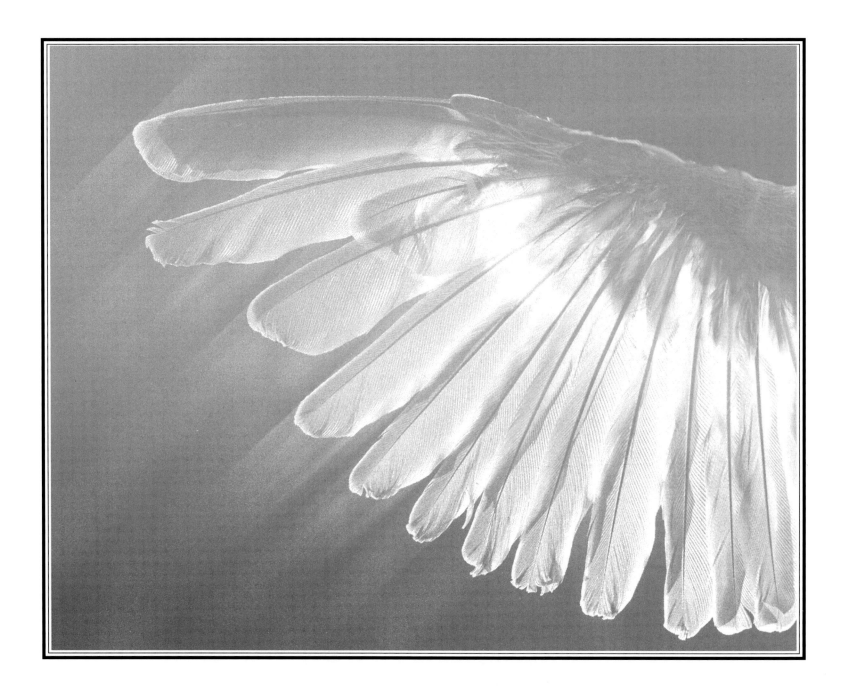

CHAPTER THIRTEEN - EYES ON THE PRIZE

"When someone you love is sick, you feel worried that the last time you spent with them will be the last time you ever spend with them. In a way, it feels scary. When that happens you can go into your imagination and see them coming home as good as new."

— John M. - 8 years old.

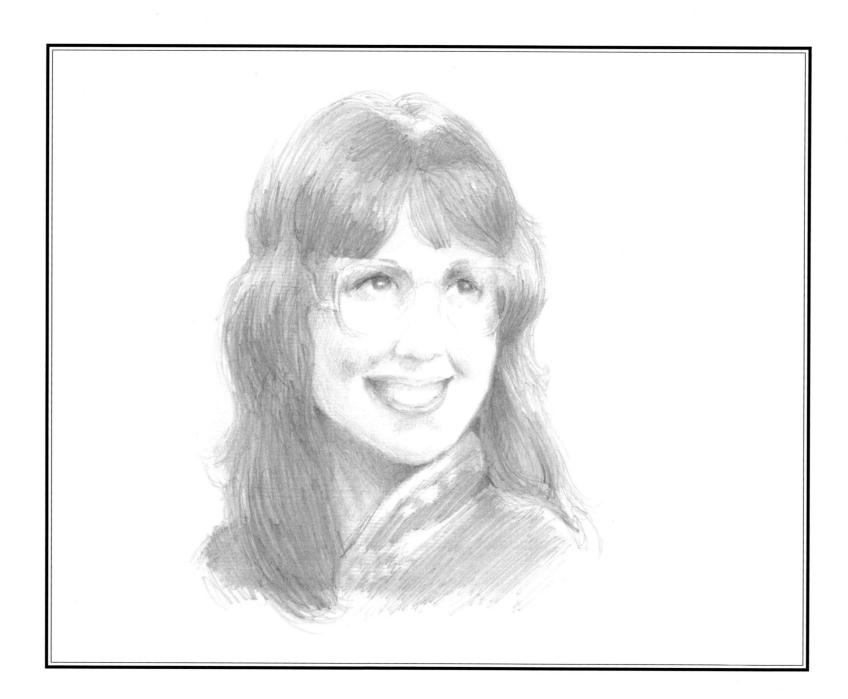

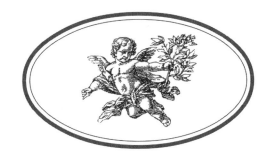

EYES ON THE PRIZE

"One kind word can warm three winter months."
—Japanese Proverb

I was invited to go on a local television program and talk about the children who have changed my life. Ken Schram, the show's host, introduced me to his studio audience. He spoke about the blessings of volunteerism and asked me to tell the audience about my experience with Darlene. I was happy to oblige. "Everyone loves to hear about Darlene," I replied as I began to tell her story.

Moving to Luxembourg was exciting for Darlene's entire family. They were making new friends and enjoying their new home and new school activities.

All this abruptly changed when the school bus driver opened the door at Darlene's stop one afternoon. As she was leaving the bus, she was struck by an approaching car. Her injuries were so severe she lapsed into unconsciousness.

She was flown back to America and brought to Children's Hospital in Seattle. At the age of fifteen, this beautiful young lady was no longer able to walk or talk. Her injuries were devastating, the doctors explained, and she lay in a kind of waking coma. The longer she remained in that state, the less likely she was to come out of it. Frankly, there was little hope for Darlene's recovery.

We met soon after she was transferred to the Miracle House. One night as she lay pale and helpless in her bed, I leaned over the bed rail and smiled into her eyes. Darlene responded with an unnatural giggle and raised her hand in a jerky motion with two fingers forming the "victory" sign.

As I looked into her dark eyes, I said to the hospital staff, "I'm not a doctor, but I can see she's still in there."

Darlene's parents were lovingly attentive throughout the entire ordeal. The weeks and months passed with no discernible change in Darlene's condition.

Every Wednesday night she was placed carefully into a long, slender cart and the two of us took off on an adventure down the hospital corridors.

One week the cart became a train speeding down the Pacific Coast to Los Angeles. The next week it was a helicopter hovering over the Grand Canyon. Yet another time it was a magic carpet dipping and turning in the skies over Washington, DC. I wheeled her up and down the hospital corridors describing the sights on our imaginary tours, always hoping to see Darlene emerge from the gray haze of her coma.

Her response remained the same, however: the unnatural giggle followed by her fingers making the "V" sign. During our escapades down the hallways people would ask, "Why do you bother talking to her like that?"

I would always answer, "I can't quite explain it, but after all of these years with the children, they have taught me how to read eyes. I can see that this young lady knows what I am saying."

The year passed in a series of Wednesday visits. One magic evening when I was making my rounds, Kitty, one of three girls who shared Darlene's room, was eager for me to get to Darlene's bed. She kept repeating, "You haven't said good night to Darlene yet."

"I will, Kitty, I will. Just a minute." Another child had just come in from surgery, and I was lingering at her bedside. But Kitty was not to be discouraged. "Pleeeease, go say good night to Darlene!"

"Okay, Kitty, okay!" Reluctantly, I left the child who was recovering from surgery and turned to Darlene. Her eyes were closed, and I thought she'd fallen asleep waiting for me to come. I felt a twinge of guilt. "Good night, Sweetheart. I'll be back to see you next week." At the sound of my voice she opened her large brown eyes and said three words, "I love you!" I was stunned. Had I actually heard what I thought I had heard? Did I imagine it? Tears filled my eyes. I said to Kitty, "You tricked me, young lady!"

Unable to contain her excitement a moment longer Kitty exclaimed, "No, Phil. Her mom came to see her last Sunday and she came out of the coma. We waited all this time to surprise you!"

Remembering Darlene's German background, I began to count, "Ein, zwei, drei."

"Vier, fünf, sechs," she answered with a sly smile. She giggled again, but this time it sounded soft, full and completely natural. I had always known she was "still in there." And now she was back!

"That's Darlene's story," I told the studio audience. "Once she was out of the coma, she continued her recovery and returned to high school. She went on to business school, got married and had two children. Then I lost track of her."

"You lost track of her, Phil," said Ken Schram, "but we've found her."

He gestured toward the back of the set. The curtains parted and Darlene, now a twenty-six-year-old woman, stepped forward into the lights. I threw my arms around her and said, "Ein, zwei, drei."

"Vier, fünf, sechs," she answered and then whispered, "I love you."

Darlene had indeed been "in there" as I had surmised on our first visit. When I looked into her eyes that first night, somehow I recognized her courage, hope, and faith, all of the qualities that would be the keys to her recovery. Darlene looked out from the depths of her devastating injury and flashed the "V" sign.

She knew that one day she would be victorious.

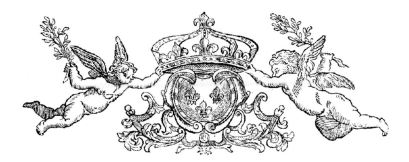

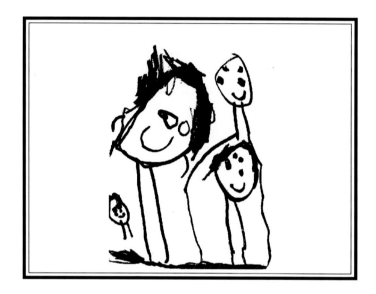

"I love to hug my mom and my dad. Everybody can be good at it.
I hug my best friend. I like to hug at bedtime. I like the book about Snow
White at bedtime. I like to play with my best friend. We go to the birthday
and play 'Put the Shoe on Cinderella.' I like Snow White. She sleeps and
sleeps and dreams. Fish sleep but they don't dream. Stars don't sleep.
But stars do dream."

— Mackenzie H. - 3 years old.

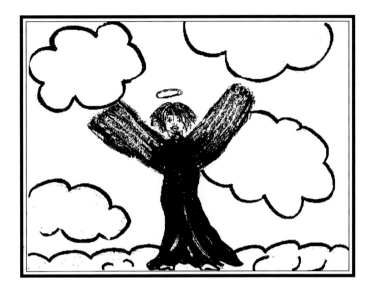

"The first time I saw an angel, it was kind of a shock because I had not seen one before. It came when I was dreaming but it was so real. It had a long dress that was made out of light. It said encouraging things. The wings were made of light in a peach color. They are encouraging you to do good things and they are protecting you and always watching over you. When the angel talks to me I feel excited and I have a weird feeling too that I can't describe. It feels good in my heart."

— Savannah S. - 8 years old.

CHAPTER FOURTEEN - FORGIVENESS

"Everybody has a heart. Even bad guys have a heart. They just don't feel the goodness inside of them and that's why they feel bad. But they are not really bad. They just don't know how to treat people."
— Lisa W. 8 years old.

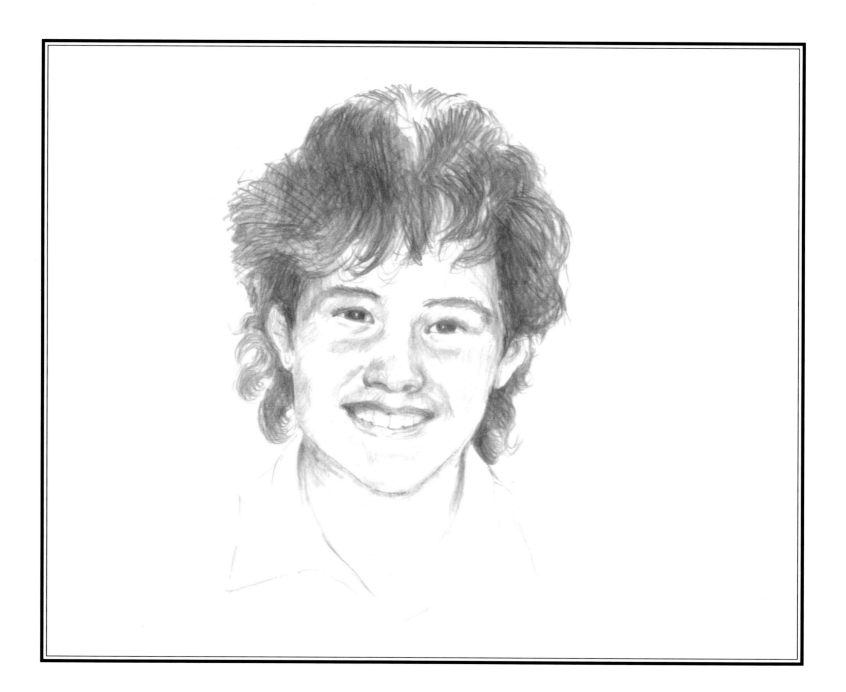

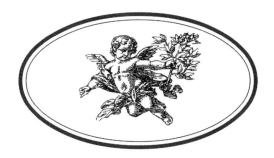

FORGIVENESS

"He who is devoid of the power to forgive is devoid of the power to love."
— Dr. Martin Luther King, Jr.

I was lost in my own thoughts when a nurse's aide approached me. "There is a young lady upstairs whom I believe you should meet. Her name is Lynn. She's fifteen years old and has cystic fibrosis."

As we walked together up the stairs, I reflected on the effects of cystic fibrosis, that insidious disease of the lungs. I wondered how it might feel to go through childhood appearing to be normal in every respect while unable to take a deep breath. The simplest of pleasures such as singing, dancing, skipping, playing jump rope, sports activities—all of these things are tremendously challenging for children with unreliable lungs.

The dark-eyed brunette sitting upright in her bed wasted not a moment before she said, "They say I have three more months to live. Do you believe them?"

I wasn't sure how to respond to such a poignant question. After pausing for a moment, I asked, "Do you believe them?"

Her animated response came bouncing across the room, "Of course not! What do you think?"

"Well, we've just met, but from that determined reply, I'm inclined to believe you!"

She was an enthusiastic open book and began reciting every chapter of her life. She had a close relationship with her family, loved to draw, and had missed so much school that graduation had become little more than a dream, but she was driven to get her GED.

Given the brutality of the disease that had ruled her life, it is remarkable that Lynn was able to retain her spunky teenage normality. Like most other girls her age, she had a best friend whom she talked to for hours, she knew every detail about a famous singer whom she idolized, she looked forward to getting her driver's license, and she longed to dance.

I loved to see her walking the halls hand in hand with her best friend, seventeen-year-old Christie. They shared their burdens and the challenges posed by the illness, but more importantly, they shared a strong personal faith and the bountiful energy of teenage conversations interspersed with musical giggles.

Lynn never ceased to surprise me. While vacationing in Maui, Helen and I were enjoying a glorious sunrise over Mount Haleakala when our solitude was interrupted by the telephone. "Sir, this is Security. You have two visitors on their way to your condo." I hurried to the front door. There she was with her mother close behind.

"Lynn, for Heaven's sake! What are you doing over here? How did you manage oxygen bottles on the airplane? How did you make the transfer in Honolulu?" I was absolutely astonished. There must have been signed releases beyond count to allow such fragile cargo to embark on this journey across the ocean.

Her reply came straight from the heart, "I wanted to see you. "The predicted "three months to live" had long since passed, and here she was, radiantly alive and on my doorstep.

A Bible verse came to mind, Mark 5:36 -- "Do not fear, only believe." It became the life line between the two of us: the ending to our phone conversations, the salutation to our letters.

Lynn combined her marvelous sense of humor and a polished artistic flair to produce wonderful cartoons. The ones she did for me were usually poking fun at "Santa." One of my favorites is: Santa in red swimming trunks on the beach in Hawaii saying, "Hang loose!" In another one has him nosing around a Christmas tree in someone's home, "Searching for the spirit of Christmas."

"Do not fear, only believe," was an appropriate quote for Lynn. She seemed to be fearless in her approach to everything she did. It was now a year and a half past her date with destiny, and she wanted to get her driver's license. She began her driving lessons with such spirited abandon that she terrified her mother and everyone else on the road in Snohomish County.

That same year, Lynn decided to learn how to play golf. She attacked the ball with vigor, the way she approached life itself. Swinging wildly at times, she expected to participate like everyone else and was impatient to exceed her previous performance at every tee. This approach often drove her to extreme fatigue and left her searching for her next breath. Her body could not sustain the energy she required of it.

When she found herself back in the hospital, I stopped in for a visit. True to form, she hit me with a blast of enthusiasm as I entered the room, "My favorite singer is doing a concert in Texas! How I wish I could see him!"

I turned to the Rotary Wishing Well, and to Lynn's delight arrangements were made for the trip to Dallas for the concert. She was almost beside herself with excitement during their departure. As her mom pushed the wheelchair up the long ramp, Lynn was waving good-bye so rapidly, I believe her fluttering hands could have propelled the plane.

Helen and I waited for their return.

"Since you get more joy out of giving joy to others, you should put a good deal of thought into the happiness that you are able to give."

—Eleanor Roosevelt

Her wheelchair was the last to leave the aircraft. Exhausted, sad, and wan, she related the concert details in muted tones. "He sang beautifully. The Rotarians arranged for me to get backstage with my wheelchair. I just sat and sat outside his dressing room door, waiting. " She held her hand in front of my face and gestured, "I was that close!" Her hand froze in the air, still measuring the distance between her thumb and forefinger. She shook her head in disbelief. An involuntary sigh escaped from her lungs. She was clearly heartbroken.

Her mother continued the story. "Finally a man appeared and said, 'Sorry, none of his fans are allowed beyond this point.' " I recreated the scene in my mind. That beautiful young girl in her wheelchair, so close to fulfilling her most coveted dream. Having sent him so many letters and photographs over the years, she may have innocently believed that he would instantly recognize her.

The sound of Lynn's voice interrupted my thoughts. She lamented, "He must not have known it was me." And with that, she forgave him.

In that instant she gave me a key to genuine forgiveness. I realized that when someone mistreats us, they simply haven't recognized who we truly are. When the tables are turned and we mistreat others, perhaps we have not recognized who they are.

My mind traveled back to World War II and a military foe I faced in North Africa. Both of us were fighting a war that began with hatreds and misunderstandings far removed from the nineteen year-old boys who were sent to fight for their countries.

My opponent was captured. When I saw that convoy of prisoners roll by me at Souk-el-Arba in Tunisia, I thought to myself, "There goes the enemy." I am certain he thought the same thing when he saw me standing beside the road.

Yet several short years later, I ended up selling Mercedes Benz cars and he ended up at the German Consulate in my home town. He bought a car from me and we became close friends.

"We have forgotten
who we are.
We ask for the gift
of remembering
...and the strength to
change.
We ask forgiveness.
We have forgotten
who we are."

— Excerpt from the United Nations Environmental Sabbath Program

I have heard it said, "I have seen the enemy and he is us." Unbeknownst to her, Lynn taught me to think about this phrase in a slightly different manner. Now that I have truly seen the enemy, I realize he is ignorance.

Summers in the Pacific Northwest can quicken your heart and fill your soul. The hills come alive in varying shades of green, and the trees clamor with the chirping of young birds trying their wings for the first time. Distant showers leave faint rainbows hanging in the air. The sun warms the steaming earth and paints lavender sunsets above the mountain ranges.

It seemed sadly ironic that during gorgeous days such as these, Lynn's condition should worsen. It was June twenty-fifth, two days before her seventeenth birthday. To cheer her up, I composed a few verses and affixed them to a nearby door so she could read them again and again at her leisure:

It has been said and proven true, there is but one and only you
Who's graced the lives of all you've met and reached each goal that you have set.
Your talents many you have shared; drawing, painting they've been paired
With smiles many, laughter ringing, hearts you've touched, spirits singing.
And so it seems it should be written, it's Lynn Michelle with whom we're smitten.

And now to you this bright June day we pause a moment just to say,
We love you greatly, and say again, thank you, charmer, for being our friend.

Over time her condition deteriorated. The unrelenting drumbeat that dictates the lives of the chronically ill marked off her remaining days. Hospital stays became longer and more frequent, her breathing became more labored, and medication provided little or no relief. Her face was pallid, and her damp hair was matted against her forehead.

I knew she could not survive much longer. Well aware that her journey toward the hereafter was drawing near, she looked into my eyes and said, "Do not fear, only believe."

She may not have been able to dance like her teenage schoolmates, but even now her eyes danced, her words danced, and her soul danced. Lynn's faith was an integral part of her personality, and she had no doubt that she would dwell in the afterlife.

Just before she died she turned to her family and said, "Do you know what I am going to do when I get there? I'm going to dance!" she declared smiling.

"I'm going to dance and dance and dance!"

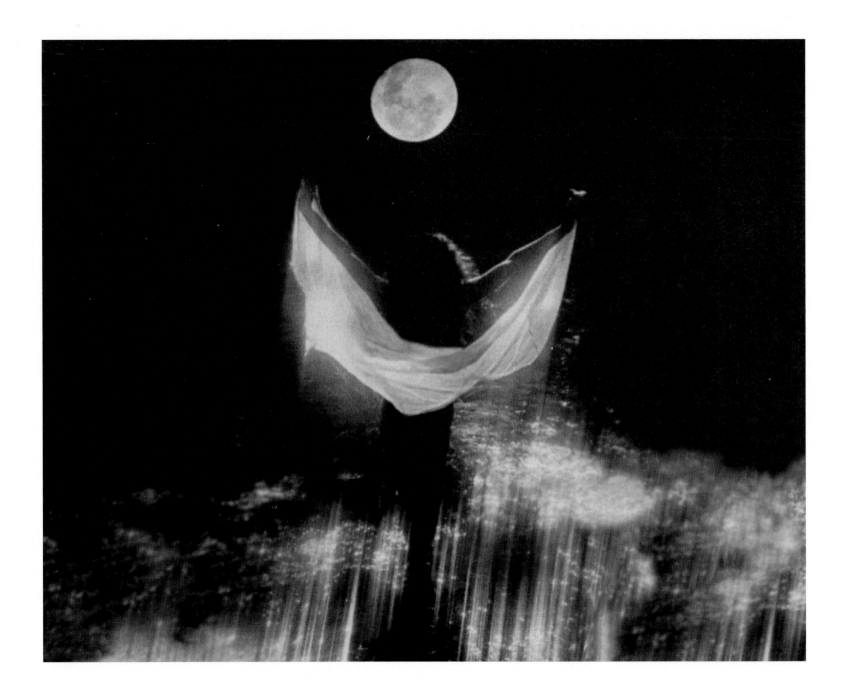

CHAPTER FIFTEEN - AN UNEXPECTED GIFT

"The earth is round, so when your spirit goes up to be with God it really doesn't go up. It could go into a lot of different directions that we don't understand because we still have our bodies on and we only know about up and down. I know it feels really good though, because my grandma died and came back and she is not a bit afraid to go again. She says it feels like flying"

— Joel P. - 9 years old.

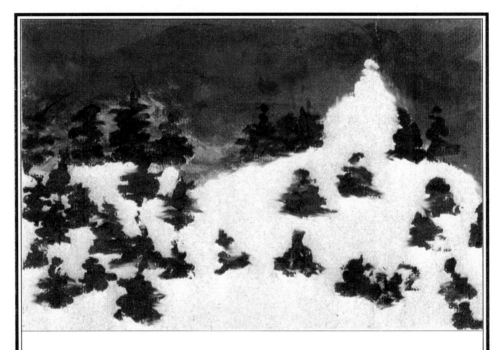

A winter landscape painted by mouth by "Blue Eyes."

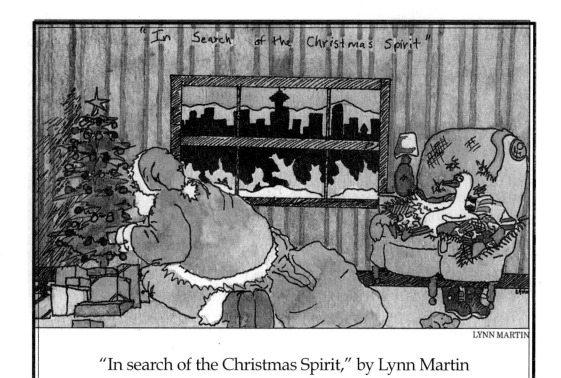

"In search of the Christmas Spirit," by Lynn Martin

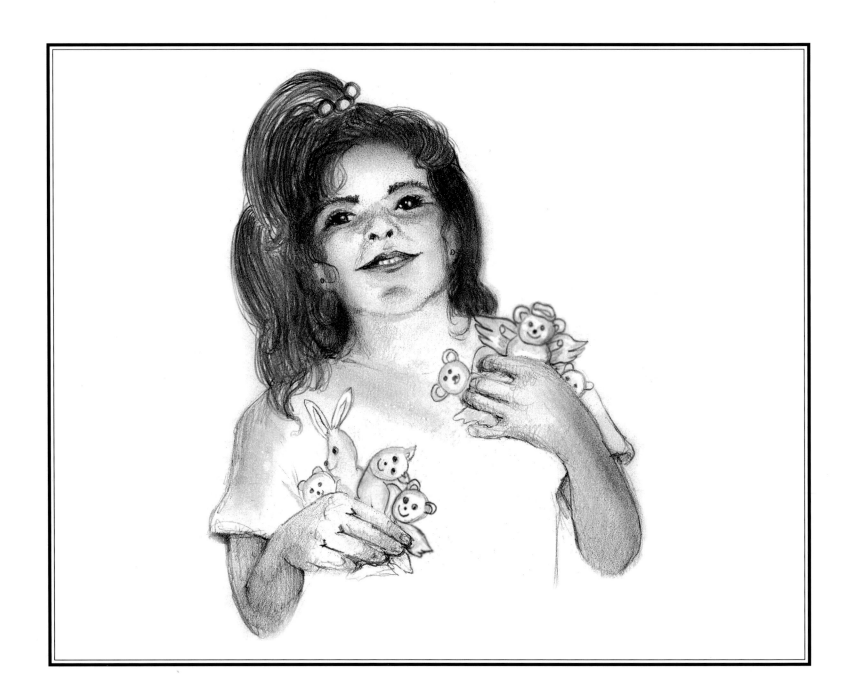

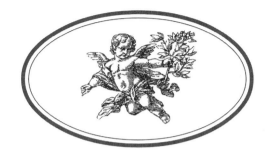

AN UNEXPECTED GIFT

"Do what you can with what you have, where you are."
— Theodore Roosevelt

From the age of three, Sherin loved to play with her stuffed animal collection. As far as she was concerned, her brightly colored bean-bag "babies" were real. Each one had a name and a distinctive personality to match. She spent hours with her babies, talking about their favorite things to do and planning their next pretend birthday parties.

By the time she was six, Sherin's family of babies had increased to over one hundred in number. Her menagerie outgrew its place on the bed and had expanded to take over every spare inch of her room. Sherin felt completely surrounded with the love of her tiny companions, particularly at night when the glow of her nightlight was reflected in their small shining eyes.

"With every

deed

you are sowing

a seed,

though

the harvest

you may not see."

—Ella Wheeler Wilcox

Once she was in school, Sherin enjoyed sitting on her bed and doing her homework with her babies. Her schooling experience brought with it new friends and a larger perspective of the world.

One day, she came home from her fourth grade class and had a serious talk with her babies. Her mother overheard her saying, "Today in school I learned about diabetes. My friend Bobby has the diabetes problem. He needs to get well, and we are going help him!"

Her mother came into the room and asked, "What were you saying about what you learned in school today?" Sherin pulled a notice from her back pack. Mom perused the leaflet and began reading aloud. "An auction for Juvenile Diabetes . . ."

Sherin interrupted, "I am going to give my babies to the auction, Mom."

"All of them?" her mother asked in disbelief.

"I really think they can help Bobby." With that, she tenderly piled her small friends into her new red wagon. The collection filled the cart to overflowing.

It was then that I received a call from the Miracle House asking, "Santa, how would you like to pick up some very special toys for the juvenile diabetes auction?"

Sherin's tiny companions fetched a high price at the auction, not only for the spirited toys themselves, but for the spirit in which they were given.

Helen and I were so moved by this young lady's generous heart that we decided to create a new tradition in her honor. During the first week of every month, Mr. and Mrs. Claus bring one hundred brightly colored, tiny stuffed animals to the Miracle House emergency room.

When Sherin told her babies they could help, they must have been thrilled with the opportunity. Several thousand of them have since found good homes in the loving arms of children who need them.

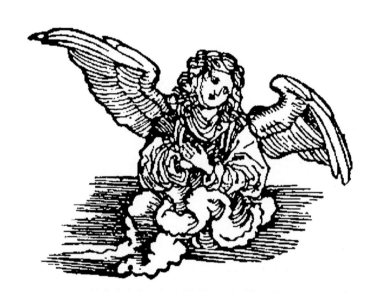

ACKNOWLEDGEMENTS

Writing a book was never in my life plans. It seemed that between commitments to family, community and work, my schedule was full. But something was missing. The stories of my life's true teachers—the special children who touched my life—needed to be told.

I want to acknowledge my family and especially our dear daughter Dianne, whom I lovingly thank for saving everything I've written since she was in the ninth grade. I run the obvious risk of overlooking someone, yet some names must be mentioned.

To my friend Bill Gates II whose foreword so sensitively and beautifully sets the tone for this book, I am deeply grateful. The Reverend Bruce Larson, Pastor Emeritus at University Presbyterian Church was my mentor and encourager when the *third eight* was born. The entire staff of Children's Hospital, but especially the RN's who embody consistency, reliability and love. They have been sentinels of hope over the decades. To the hospital itself, never swaying in its mission to provide uncompromising pediatric care, regardless of a family's ability to pay. This outstanding house of miracles has been a revered beacon of empathy and healing. I trust the reader will also sense its devotion within these pages.

I thank the Roots & Wings Society staff and Board of Trustees whose vision has brought *Angels Among Us* into print. Alison Asher, its founder, helped me write these stories as they appear in this book. She continues to be a guiding light without peer.

Of course, my hundreds of young teachers at Children's must be thanked, especially these twenty-four: Boris, Kitty, Kathy, Terry, Beth, Little Joe, Angie, David, Lynn, Ross, Doug, Mark, Connor, Bobbie, Adam, Christie, Courtney, Stephanie, Gracie, Shannon, B.J., Aaron, Patrick, and loyal Jimmy who came in his wheelchair and brought Santa a gift every Christmas for the past eighteen years. In honor of these children I pray that as we close the pages of this book, we will open our hearts forevermore to the life-lessons taught by these young angels among us.

And finally, to my beloved wife and partner Helen. Through it all, her loyalty and support has never wavered. Her love—constant and encouraging—has been a life ring of survival no matter the family situation or business challenge.

ABOUT THE AUTHOR

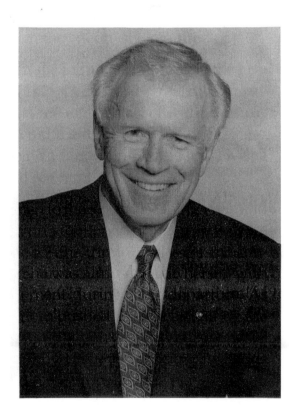

Phil Smart was born and raised in the Pacific Northwest and has been a resident of Seattle since 1920. He became an Eagle Scout during his adolescence and continued as Scoutmaster for fourteen years as an adult. During the Second World War he served under General George Patton.

He has been active in community service for more than fifty years including his tenure as a ward volunteer at Children's Hospital and Regional Medical Center. He has appeared on television and inspired audiences large and small to contribute their gift of time. Phil is married to Helen, his bride of sixty years. They live in Seattle, Washington where they enjoy their children, grandchildren and great grandchildren.

To Order Additional Books From Roots & Wings

Telephone Orders: 1-800-273-4591 or (206) 780-0488
Please have your credit card ready.

ON-LINE ORDERS: www.roots ‑ wings.com FAX: (206) 780-0489

Please send me _____ copies of *Angels Among Us* ($21.00 each)

Please send me _____ copies of *Soaring Into The Storm* ($21.00 each)
$5.00 handling fee plus shipping charges.

Date: ___/___/___ Phone: _____ Fax or Email _____

Name: _____

Shipping Address: _____

City: _____ State _____ Zip: _____

Payment: ❑ Check   ❑ Visa   ❑ MasterCard

Card number: _____

Name on card: _____ Exp. date: _____

MAIL ORDERS: PO BOX 11808 BAINBRIDGE ISLAND WA. 98110

If you are shipping in Washington State please add 8.8% sales tax.

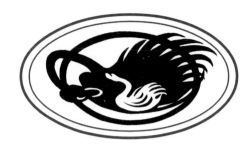

The Roots & Wings Society
Providing comfort and guidance to families overcoming adversity

100% of net royalties from this book provide medical services for children.

We all face unforeseen storms in our lives. Sometimes the outcomes can be devastating. When we lose a home to a natural disaster, a family member suddenly becomes seriously ill, or violent crime leaves its mark on a child, the entire family is in need of comfort and guidance. Each book we publish gathers the wisdom of ordinary extraordinary people from around the world who have overcome adversity. Our books offer that wisdom in a manner that is clear and simple enough for all family members to understand. Through the success of our first publication, *Soaring into the Storm*, we have been invited into the innermost hearts of those whom we may never meet, from one corner of the globe to the other.

In the darkest night of the soul
the written word is welcome where no other companion dares to tread.
This is truly sacred ground.

The Roots & Wings Society is a nonprofit, tax exempt organization. We are seeking corporate sponsors to help us provide thousands of books to families who are recovering from life's most difficult passages, including recovery from: violent crime, loss of a loved one, natural disasters, and war.
www.roots-wings.com 1-800-273-4591